An Introduction to
Child and Adolescent
Mental Health

SAGE has been part of the global academic community since 1965, supporting high quality research and learning that transforms society and our understanding of individuals, groups and cultures. SAGE is the independent, innovative, natural home for authors, editors and societies who share our commitment and passion for the social sciences.

Find out more at: **www.sagepublications.com**

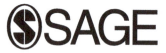

An Introduction to
Child and **Adolescent**
Mental Health

Maddie Burton, Erica Pavord and Briony Williams

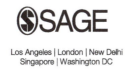

Los Angeles | London | New Delhi
Singapore | Washington DC

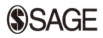

Los Angeles | London | New Delhi
Singapore | Washington DC

SAGE Publications Ltd
1 Oliver's Yard
55 City Road
London EC1Y 1SP

SAGE Publications Inc.
2455 Teller Road
Thousand Oaks, California 91320

SAGE Publications India Pvt Ltd
B 1/I 1 Mohan Cooperative Industrial Area
Mathura Road
New Delhi 110 044

SAGE Publications Asia-Pacific Pte Ltd
3 Church Street
#10-04 Samsung Hub
Singapore 049483

Editor: Becky Taylor
Associate editor: Emma Milman
Production editor: Katie Forsythe
Copyeditor: Jane Fricker
Proofreader: Rose James
Indexer: William Farrington
Marketing manager: Tamara Navaratnam
Cover design: Naomi Robinson
Typeset by: C&M Digitals (P) Ltd, Chennai, India

Library of Congress Control Number: 2014933386

British Library Cataloguing in Publication data

A catalogue record for this book is available from
the British Library

ISBN 978-1-4462-4944-4
ISBN 978-1-4462-4945-1 (pbk)

CONTENTS

ABOUT THE AUTHORS

Maddie Burton is a Registered Mental Health Nurse and for several years worked in both inpatient (Tier 4) and community (Tiers 2, 3) CAMH services. Maddie joined the University of Worcester in 2009 as Senior Lecturer Child and Adolescent Mental Health and maintains close links with practice in the CAMHS. Maddie holds membership of the Association for Child and Adolescent Mental Health and the Association for Infant Mental Health. She is a Fellow of the Higher Education Academy.

Erica Pavord has worked as a counsellor for children, young people and families for Face to Face which is part of Monmouthshire Youth Service since 2007. She works in a variety of settings – a secondary school, a GP practice and youth centres – offering one-to-one talking therapy, therapeutic play and family counselling. She also works with the CAMH Family Therapy service in Monmouthshire. She trained initially as an integrative counsellor and then as a systemic practitioner. Before becoming a counsellor, Erica worked for 16 years as English teacher in secondary schools in London, East Africa and South Wales. She started bringing together the two parts of her career in 2010 when she became a sessional lecturer at the University of Worcester as part of the Foundation Degree team. She recently started teaching a CAMH module as a Visiting Lecturer on the BA Education at the University of South Wales.

Briony Williams initially trained as an Occupational Therapist and worked in a variety of mental health settings including substance misuse, in patients and community mental health. She moved to Coventry University as a Lecturer Practitioner in 1999 and then worked full time for several years as Admissions Tutor for the Occupational Therapy course. Briony wrote the Foundation Degree in Child and Adolescent Mental Health at University of Worcester in 2007 in collaboration with clinicians working in Child and Adolescent Mental Health services. She had an honorary contract with the Early Intervention for Psychosis Service in Worcester. She now manages a team in the Health and Applied Social Science Academic Unit in the Institute of Health and Society and also manages the McClelland Wellbeing Centre at University of Worcester.

ACKNOWLEDGEMENTS

We would like to remember our colleague Mark Prever who sadly and suddenly died in 2013. Mark taught on the Child and Adolescent Mental Health Foundation Degree. He illuminated and inspired us and the students said he was 'the best ever'. Mark's ideas around the importance of personal development and self-reflection for people working with children have influenced the content of this book. His publications on supporting children and young people will continue to inspire students on our course.

INTRODUCTION

The book is aimed at people working with children and young people and those studying related courses. This could include students and professionals in educational, health and social care settings such as schools, preschools, children's centres, looked after children's sector, youth work and youth justice, to name a few. Those working with children, young people and families have considerable potential for thinking about and developing a deeper awareness and understanding of child and adolescent mental health.

'Mental Health is Everyone's Business' is the coalition government's mental health strategy launched in 2011. With costs to the economy of over £105 billion and more importantly an emotional cost for individuals and families, addressing the mental health needs of the population at the earliest possible opportunity is a necessity. Half of lifetime mental health problems begin to emerge by age 14 and three-quarters by the mid-twenties (Department of Health, 2011). Workers in Early Years, schools, colleges, youth services, health and any setting where there are children, young people and families would benefit from increasing their knowledge and understanding of child and adolescent mental health. Workers need to be able to respond in a supportive and timely fashion and refer appropriately when needed.

The book gives a comprehensive overview of the key issues in child and adolescent mental health. The authors are involved in the provision of studies at the University of Worcester. The choice of chapters was influenced by the content of the programme.

There are three main sections within the book. The first section concentrates on developing an understanding of child and adolescent mental health conditions; supported by the contextual role of infant, child and adolescent development and safeguarding and children's rights. The next section looks at ways of working with children, young people and families. It includes working with mental health promotion strategies, interpersonal skills and therapeutic communication, interventions in child and adolescent mental health and working in groups.

The final section of the book includes values and attitudes when working with children and young people. The section concentrates on individuals and the wider role and impact of society.

The book will present complex theories and ideas in a clear, accessible and user-friendly way that is practical and interactive. Throughout the chapters there will be distinct activities, reflection and discussion points, scenario case studies and vignettes. The case studies and vignettes have been adapted from practice or are from personal experiences and published literature. For the purposes of anonymity names and any identifying information has been changed.

REFERENCES

Department of Health (2011) *No Health without Mental Health: A Cross Government Mental Health Outcomes Strategy for People of all Ages*. Available from: www.dh.gov.uk/en/Publicationsandstatistics/Publications/PublicationsPolicyAndGuidance/DH_123766 (accessed August 2012).

1

CHILDREN AND YOUNG PEOPLE'S MENTAL HEALTH

MADDIE BURTON

Overview

- Child and adolescent mental health – strategic view
- Child and adolescent mental health – context today
- Defining child and adolescent mental health
- Theoretical models
- Risk and resilience
- Mental health conditions:
  - Depression
  - Anxiety
  - Self-harm
  - Suicidal behaviour
  - Eating disorders
  - Early onset psychosis and substance misuse
  - Emerging personality disorder
- Neuro-developmental conditions

INTRODUCTION

This chapter will provide an overview of child and adolescent mental health problems and services. Psychological, biological, social and environmental theories inform our understanding of mental health problems. It is generally understood that a combination of *nature* and *nurture* theories, used to inform an understanding of human development, also offer the most likely theoretical explanations for understanding child and adolescent mental health. It is about the inter-play and inter-relation between:

- Biological factors (brain development and genetics);
- Psychological variables such as coping mechanisms;
- Genetic and physiological characteristics;
- Environmental circumstances (positive or negative).

Another way of thinking about this is that an individual's inherent genes are triggered by experiences in childhood. Alternatively, positive experiences can mitigate or offset genetic factors. The nature and process of risk and resilience theory also requires exploration in order to understand the complex interplay between all these theoretical models. Child and adolescent mental health encompasses a large area and it is difficult to fully explore them all within the confines of a chapter; so some areas have a larger focus here than others.

CHILD AND ADOLESCENT MENTAL HEALTH: A STRATEGIC VIEW

Child and adolescent mental health is a relatively new psychiatric healthcare specialism; the Child and Adolescent Mental Health Services (CAMHS) we have today were commissioned and established following the *Together We Stand* Health Advisory Service Report (1995). Prior to that date child psychiatry was commonly situated in Child Guidance Clinics or Child Behaviour Clinics, with children being typically referred with symptoms such as larceny, masturbation and conduct disorder. Child Guidance Clinics were based on local commitment rather than explicit government policy. Young people with conditions including eating disorders and psychosis were treated in adult in-patient psychiatric hospitals and units. Since 2010 hospital mangers now have an obligation to provide age appropriate facilities (Barber et al., 2012).

Current CAMHS provision as established in 1995 includes a tiered strategic service:

Tier 1: a primary level of care; professionals include:

- GPs
- Health visitors
- School nurses
- Social workers
- Teachers
- Juvenile justice workers
- Voluntary agencies
- Social services.

Tier 2: a service provided by professionals relating to workers in primary care; professionals include:

- Clinical child psychologists
- Paediatricians (especially community)
- Educational psychologists
- Child and adolescent psychiatrists
- Child and adolescent psychotherapists
- Community nurses/nurse specialists
- Family therapists.

Tier 3: a specialised service for more severe, complex or persistent disorders; professionals include:

- Child and adolescent psychiatrists
- Clinical child psychologists
- Nurses (community or in-patient)
- Child psychotherapists
- Occupational therapists
- Speech and language therapists
- Art, music and drama therapists
- Family therapists.

Tier 4: essential tertiary level services such as day units, highly specialised out-patient teams and in-patient units. All of the above Tier 3 professionals would be included in this tier.

CHILD AND ADOLESCENT MENTAL HEALTH TODAY

Many mental health problems have origins in childhood (Dogra et al., 2009). Half of lifetime mental health problems (excluding dementia) begin to emerge by age 14 and three-quarters by the mid-twenties (Department of Health, 2011a). The prevalence of many childhood mental health disorders has increased in the western world during the last 25 years, particularly conduct disorders, anxiety and depression (Street et al., 2007).

Ten per cent of five to fifteen year olds have a diagnosable mental health disorder. This suggests that around 1.1 million children and young people under eighteen would benefit from specialist services. There are up to 45,000 young people with a severe mental health disorder. Around forty per cent of children with a mental health disorder are not currently receiving any specialist service. (DH and DE, 2004: Rationale 2.2)

Activity

Why do you think there is an increase in reports of mental health problems for children and young people in Britain today?

There is a mixed picture of theories with no definitive answers! There is increased recognition and alertness to the possibility of mental health problems. Mental health is now perhaps considered as an explanation and understanding of presenting behaviours. The mental health agenda is now much more publicised than previously, in part due to the media and to government health awareness programmes. This has led to a more open discourse and together with all other health issues information is now much more readily available via the internet. Both parents and children are in some cases more likely to ask for help than in the past. Some Early Years settings professionals are now taking more interest in emotional and mental health. Children's centres which began with Sure Start in the last decade are paying more attention and recognising the significance of poor emotional and mental health in children, their carers and families. They have instigated active programmes and links with health care professionals such as health visitors and local child and adolescent Tier 2 and 3 services. The Healthy Child Programme: Pregnancy and the First Five Years of Life (Department of Health, 2009) has a strong emphasis and commitment to improving attachment quality between parents and children, a strong indicator of the now recognised importance of attachment and improved social and emotional wellbeing. Early Years, teacher training programmes and social work training are rather slower in catching up with infant, child and adolescent mental health issues and understanding, as integral parts of their training. It is unfortunately at the moment patchy and in some areas non-existent. However the health driven agenda has raised awareness in education settings with programmes such as the three-year Targeted Mental Health in Schools (TaMHS) from 2008 to 2011 (Chimat, 2012), although this was a trial in specific areas in the country and only covered the 5–13 age group. Other initiatives have included Social and Emotional Aspects of Learning (SEAL, 2010) and Personal, Social and Health Education (PSHE, 2011).

CONTEXT OF CHILD AND ADOLESCENT MENTAL HEALTH

Science now evidences that infants are not too young to experience mental health problems. Those who have experienced significant maltreatment exhibit clinical symptoms of post-traumatic stress disorder (PTSD) (National Scientific Council on the Developing Child, 2004: 3). How these difficulties can be ameliorated does however offer hope for repair and will be discussed in Chapter 6.

Mental ill health is an interpretation of illness and the medicalisation of behaviours considered to be beyond the norm. What we are often presented with is a set of behaviours which could be seen to be *acting out* of the individual internal working model. So behaviours can be understood from a psychological perspective rather than a tendency for an interpretation of illness as such. Acting out is a process which aims to get the hurt addressed and is a defence mechanism (see Chapter 2), defending one from anxiety. Acting out is an emotional and externally visible response to feelings which are unmanageable.

Children and young people referred to CAMHS at Tier 2 and above are always thought about systemically; within their current and previous contexts of family or carers and including other systems around the child or young person, such as educational and community settings. It is important for all those working with children and young people throughout all tiers to be mindful of the child or young person's context. Professionals and clinicians will be attentive in history taking a full developmental history of the individual and the family beginning at a point prior to conception. Almost always a history provides the clues with which to help understanding of behaviours and other presentations.

A diagnosis of conditions would be agreed, for example the signs and symptoms recognised in depression and eating disorders. Any condition has been with a child or young person for a relatively shorter time period than if the condition was presenting for the first time in adulthood. There is an important window of opportunity for intervention which would ideally be systemic and include the system around the child. The resulting changes brought about by interventions have more chance of success and for changes to be successful before the condition exacerbates, continuing into adulthood and becoming more concrete and difficult to treat.

One of the differences between a CAMHS and adult mental health model is that CAMHS is always a combination of medical and psychological interpretations and interventions, whereas an adult mental health model has been primarily medical in both interpretation and intervention. It is also relevant at this point to state that only GPs (although this is now less likely), and child and adolescent psychiatrists make clinical diagnoses. So it is important for children and young people where there are concerns over their mental health to be referred to a Tier 2 or 3 CAMHS team for a thorough assessment.

DEFINING CHILDREN AND YOUNG PEOPLE'S MENTAL HEALTH

Mental health is a broad concept, culturally determined, which can be complicated to interpret. It is also important to remember that meanings around mental health are culture bound and are subject to change. Universally it includes freedom from persistent problems with emotions, behaviour and social relationships (Kurtz, 1992, cited in *Together We Stand*, 1995: 18).

Mental health is aptly defined for children and young people by Hill (cited in *Together We Stand*, 1995: 15) as:

Not being easy to maintain within a context of ever changing circumstances and events which are dependent on individual potential and experience. It involves the capacity to develop in the following areas:

- Physically, emotionally, intellectually and spiritually
- The ability to initiate, develop and sustain mutually satisfying personal relationships
- The ability to become aware of others and empathise with them
- The ability to use psychological distress as a developmental process, so that it does not hinder or impair further development.

In children and young people mental health is more specifically indicated by:

- A capacity to enter into and sustain mutually satisfying personal relationships.
- Continuing progression of psychological development.
- An ability to play and learn so that attainments are appropriate for age and intellectual level.
- A developing moral sense of right and wrong.
- The degree of psychological distress and maladaptive behaviour being within normal limits for the child's age and context.

Examples of potential mental health problems would include somatising features (physical symptoms with psychological origins) such as headaches, enuresis and encopresis (faecal soiling), tummy aches and sleep disturbances, self-harm, suicidal behaviours, risk taking, mood changes, behaviour changes, relationship and attachment difficulties, substance misuse, changed eating patterns, isolation and social withdrawal.

Examples of mental illness/disorder include eating disorders, anxiety disorders, depression, psychosis, conduct disorder, neuro-developmental conditions, such as attention deficit hyperactivity disorder (ADHD) and autistic spectrum disorders (ASD) – although it is now considered more appropriate to use the term autistic spectrum conditions (ASC) – developmental disorder, habit disorder, post-traumatic stress disorder and somatic disorders.

Mental health problems are relatively common but include mental health disorders, as above, which tend to be more persistent. There is a considerable overlap across the range, with 'emotional' being an element throughout. Severity and impact can span a wide range. Some children have both physical illness and mental health problems combined. For example a young person with diabetes may place themselves at risk of complications through non-compliance with treatment. Terminology such as 'disorder' can feel quite stigmatising, however it is important to recognise children and young people who may be experiencing problems, so that appropriate interventions can be organised.

All presentations also need to be thought of in the context of normal development, which is on a continuum of constant change. Any of the above illnesses and disorders can either lead to or be associated with other behaviours and problems. For example conduct disorder may precede substance misuse. It is important to remember that risk taking behaviours and mood changes are thought of as normal in adolescent behaviour. Potential symptoms need to be considered from a developmental perspective but also the context of the child or young person.

However many significantly impaired children do not meet diagnostic criteria or they meet symptomatic criteria but they are not impaired. It is about making a clinical judgement regarding diagnosis. Diagnosis is about bringing together illnesses with the same features although most 'disorders' are multi-factorial in causation. Diagnosis is about symptoms and signs of a disorder but not necessarily about treatment, although it helps inform treatment choices.

THEORETICAL MODELS

The different theoretical models used to understand and interpret an individual's presenting features of mental ill health consist of several overlapping and interrelated domains including:

> *Medical or biological theory:* illness is determined by an individual's genetic make-up. Illness is classified according to ICD 10 and DSM 5. Traditionally adult mental health is more firmly positioned here.

> *Psychological theory:* cognitive and emotional factors including attachment theory. Insecure attachment can increase risks to mental health in infants, children and adolescents and throughout the life span (World Health Organization, 2012). Secure attachment (Bowlby, 2008 [1988]) leads to feelings of safety being internalised whereas disorganised attachment (Main and Solomon, 1986) leaves the individual with nothing to draw on in terms of a safe internal working model, with external experiences having an enduring significance throughout life.

> *Systemic, social and environmental theories:* the impact of context – family stressors, poor social support, poverty, housing, income, parenting style, parental mental health, cultural influence, peer rejection and stressful life events including bereavement and loss. Relationship patterns and links between family members need to be considered as these will be relevant to informing understanding; also areas of parental conflict, quality of sibling relationships, the relationship of both parents with the child and the parents' own early experiences, or as aptly described by Karr-Morse and Wiley (1997), the 'ghosts from the nursery'.

RISK AND RESILIENCE MODEL

The risk and resilience model was identified by Pearce (1993, cited in *Together We Stand*, 1995). He defined three areas of risk which were: environmental/contextual, the family and the young person/child as follows:

Environmental/contextual

- Socioeconomic disadvantage
- Homelessness
- Disaster
- Discrimination
- Violence in the community
- Being a refugee/asylum seeker
- Other significant life event.

Family

- Early attachment/nurturing problems
- Parental conflict
- Family breakdown
- Inconsistent/unclear discipline
- Hostile and/or rejecting relationships
- Significant adults' failure to adapt to child's changing developmental needs
- Physical, emotional, sexual abuse
- Parental mental and/or physical illness
- Parental criminal behaviour
- Death and loss, bereavement issues relating to family members or friends.

Child/young person

- Genetic influences
- Low IQ or learning difficulties
- Specific developmental delay
- Communication difficulties
- Difficult temperament
- Gender identity conflict
- Chronic physical illness
- Neurological disorder
- Academic failure/poor school attendance
- Low self-esteem.

Resilience factors as identified by Pearce (1993, cited in *Together We Stand*, 1995) are as follows:

Resilience factors

- Secure attachments
- Self-esteem

- Social skills
- Familial compassion and warmth
- A stable family environment
- Social support systems that encourage personal development and coping skills
- A skill or talent.

Activity: risk and resilience model

Take a look at the case study below and consider which area of risk is evident. Are there any potential resilience or protective factors?

Jane is 14. Her grandmother has taken her to the GP. She has been feeling low and tearful for several months.

This started after losing the family home. After years of domestic violence towards Jane's mum from her partner they shared the house with, Jane's mum was courageous enough to insist he leave the family home. With him left the financial support and Jane's mum was no longer able to afford the mortgage repayments and lost the house. They lived in Bed and Breakfast for several weeks and then moved to a one bedroom flat. One of their dogs had to be given away; a neighbour took the other dog. There was no space at the B&B or provision for pets. Most personal possessions were lost; Jane left her home with the only possessions she could fit into a bin bag. Jane feels they have lost everything and feels guilty about it; she was using the phone a lot and ran up some big bills. Jane does not want to talk to her mother as her mother is depressed.

She is crying herself to sleep, not sleeping well and waking frequently. Appetite is poor and she is hardly eating anything. Sometimes she says it hurts so much inside she does not know what to do and has cut herself at times and spends a lot of time usually in her room. Prior to these events Jane won a literary award prize for story telling in the 11–13 years category in a schools competition. Now Jane has secret books where she is drawing lots of sad and angry pictures. On one of the pages she has drawn a gravestone for herself and her dog and has written 'I wish I wasn't here'. School work has started to be affected as she cannot be bothered to do anything.

Areas of evident risk for Jane

Family: Mum has *mental health problems* (clinically depressed). There has been *parental conflict and violence*. *Loss* in terms of Jane's pet dog (she'd had him since he was a puppy) and *loss* of her home.

Environment/context: *Homeless, socioeconomic disadvantage, significant life events.*

Child/young person: *Genetic influences* (parent with mental health problems), *school work* now affected.

(Continued)

(Continued)

Resilience and protective factors for Jane: Mum has modelled that she will no longer tolerate an abusive partner and has taken an active step to break the cycle of violence even though this has led to her and Jane losing their home. Clearly Jane has a *skill* or a *talent* for writing demonstrated by her literary prize.

Despite major adversity and overwhelming odds, many young people cope well. The key is *resilience*, which acts as a protective factor. Rutter (1985, 2006) described this as a dynamic evolving process and not just about static factors. The model of risk and resilience is not based on risk and protective factors in themselves but rather on how they interact. The emphasis is on the process of resilience across developmental pathways. Some young people may tick all the boxes in relation to risk factors being present early on in life. Multiple family transitions can increase risk with a cumulative effect on educational achievement, behaviour and relationships in general.

Identifying a skill or a talent as cited above should not be underestimated. Mo Farah the Olympic champion was a migrant from Somalia, escaping the civil war and arriving in London aged 8 and speaking very little English. His potential athletic talent was spotted by his PE teacher and the rest is history. The story had the potential to be so different.

It is relevant to consider strategies for promoting resilience and it has to be remembered that resilience can only develop through some exposure to risk or stress. Prior to Pearce (1993, cited in *Together We Stand*, 1995), Rutter (1985) identified that resilience develops through exposure to risk or stress at a *manageable level of intensity* at developmental points where protective factors can operate. The major risk factors for children and young people tend to operate within chronic and transitional events such as continuing family conflict, chronic and persistent bullying, long-term poverty and multiple school and home changes. Children and young people seem to show greater resilience when faced with more single one-off acute risk and adversity events, such as bereavement (Coleman and Hagell, 2007). Promoting resilience and reducing a child's exposure to risk is an important consideration. Newman (2004, cited in Coleman and Hagell, 2007: 14) suggests a three-point strategy approach:

- *Strategy one:* reduce the child's exposure to risk: school meals, after school clubs for children with no alternative but to play on the street.
- *Strategy two:* interrupt the chain reaction of negative events; if one risk factor increases others will probably follow.
- *Strategy three:* offer the child or young person positive experiences: ways of enhancing self-esteem and developing relationships with positive adults.

Highly targeted therapeutic and educational support is required for identified at risk groups including, for example, looked after children (Schofield et al., 2012). There were over 67,000 children looked after by local authorities in England as of March

2012 (Department for Education, 2013). Given such significant numbers this is a huge task. Looked after children and care leavers have a five-fold increased risk of mental, emotional and behavioural problems and a six- to seven-fold increased risk of conduct disorders (Department of Health, 2011a). A good care giving relationship can act as a protective factor and can mitigate other social and environmental factors such as poverty and disability.

For young people in the secure estate (young offender institutions) figures are even more alarming, with 29% of adolescent girls diagnosed with major depression (four to five times higher than general youth population), and 10.6% of adolescent boys diagnosed with major depression. The incidence of young people with psychosis is 10 times higher than the general population. With one in 10 boys and one in five girls having a diagnosis of ADHD, which equates to 10 to 20 times higher for girls in detention and five times higher for boys in detention than the general adolescent population (Fazel, 2008). Figures published by the Department of Health (2011b) state that since January 2002, six young people in the secure estate have killed themselves.

CLASSIFICATION SYSTEMS

There are different definitions for mental ill health. Terms such as mental disorders, mental illness and mental health problems are used interchangeably. Disorders and illness tend to include those defined by the *International Classification of Diseases* (ICD 10; World Health Organisation, 2013) – ICD 11 is due for completion by 2015 – and the *Diagnostic and Statistical Manual* (DSM 5) published in 2013 (American Psychiatric Association, 2013). Disorders include emotional, conduct and hyperkinetic (neuro-developmental). Mental health problems include a broad range of conditions and presentations which tend to also include emotional and behavioural presentations (British Medical Association Board of Science, 2006; Dogra and Leighton, 2009: 9). Variations in behaviour can be defined by ICD 10 and DSM 5 whereas behavioural symptoms can also be differently understood within a context of human experience and relationships, particularly the family.

SIGNIFICANT MENTAL HEALTH CONDITIONS

Depression

Depression was once thought to be limited to adults. Children and young people were overlooked in the past. Children who were taken to behaviour clinics may have suffered from depression but clinicians did not take notice or ask children about their feelings and moods. Kendall (2000) agrees that quiet, withdrawn children were and can often be ignored.

Childhood depression is linked with a range of negative outcomes including: impaired social adjustment, academic difficulties and increased risk of suicide.

Depression is a risk factor in suicide, and undiagnosed or untreated depression can heighten that risk. Depression is now recognised as a major public health problem in the UK and worldwide. It accounts for 15% of all disability in high-income countries. In England one in six adults and one in 20 children and young people at any one time are affected by depression and related conditions, such as anxiety. Up to 80% of adults with depression and anxiety disorders first experience them before the age of 18 (Department of Health, 2011a).

According to ICD 10 and DSM 5, depression is characterised by an episodic disorder of varying degrees of severity with depressed mood and loss of enjoyment persisting for several weeks. There must also be a presence of other symptoms including: depressive thinking, pessimism about the future, suicidal ideas and biological symptoms such as early waking, weight loss and reduced appetite (Harrington, 2003).

The criteria are similar for children and adults but with important differences (Keenan and Evans, 2009). With children and young people developmental perspectives are highly relevant. For example, eating and sleeping disturbances often present as potential symptoms, but these would be common in childhood anyway. Tearfulness and crying have a very different meaning and incidence in childhood compared with adulthood. It is also common to feel depressed. It is also important to 'normalise' sadness as a passing human condition. If sadness became persistent over time this would be different.

There are gender differences beginning in puberty and continuing into adulthood, with higher prevalence in females than males. Clear determinants are far from established (Piccinelli and Wilkinson, 2000). There may be a link to the fact of girls tending to internalise stress and boys externalising stress. Together with biological and hormonal differences there is a likelihood of more conduct and behavioural problems with boys and depressive, anxiety symptoms and eating disorders in girls.

Teenage mums experience higher rates of depression, being three times more likely to experience postnatal depression and to experience poor mental health for up to three years after the birth (Department of Health, 2007), a reminder of the nature and nurture debate and the implications for these infants and their psychological and emotional development.

Anxiety

Emotional development is a challenge for all human beings. In practice, *fears* and *anxieties* are frequently intermingled. Anxiety can be considered either normal or abnormal depending on the context and degree of the anxiety. It is an essential emotion protecting us from danger. Reasonable levels of anxiety help us to function; think of the last minute rush to hand in assignments if you are a student, or meet deadlines, or even get to school and work on time and run for the bus. Interestingly, Pearce (2004) points out that the word anxious resembles the Latin word *angre* and is the origin for the word anger, which suggests a link between anxiety and anger. Conduct disorders often operate in conjunction co-morbidly with anxiety and anger may form a link between anxiety and depression. Anxiety becomes pathological when the fear is out of proportion to the context of the life situation and, in childhood, when it is out of keeping with the expected behaviour for the developmental stage of the child (Lask, 2003). Fear is feeling a sense of threat in the presence of a particular person, situation, or object. Anxiety is a feeling of threat experienced in anticipation of an undesirable event even if the specific nature of what may happen is not known.

For example, separation anxiety would be considered normal for infants (leaving a primary carer) but less so for a teenager. In a relatively short time span, in comparison to the full length of human life, children move from a state of limited emotional understanding to becoming complex individuals. The number and complexity of emotional experiences together with modulation of human expression increase with age. It is therefore not surprising that some children and young people are easily overwhelmed and experience emotional disorders, which if they persist are debilitating and require intervention. There are *different fears for different years*. In infancy if secure attachment is accomplished fear of separation from care giver diminishes. Separation anxiety usually begins in the preschool years any time after the attachment period but typically in late childhood or early adolescence. Other fear such as the dark and then as the imagination develops ghosts and monsters can appear. Animal phobias such as a fear of spiders or dogs usually begin in childhood. Performance anxiety can emerge in late childhood and social anxiety in adolescence. Fears and anxieties are normal developmental challenges facing the maturing individual. During adolescence autonomy and independence are major developmental challenges, endeavouring to balance between compliance with rules and expressing independent autonomy. It is normal to experience conflict at some level, but the challenge posed by emerging autonomy can trigger or exacerbate interpersonal problems that require negotiation with the accompanying anxiety.

There are many variations of anxiety and the accompanying symptomatic presentations. The common underlying factor throughout differing presentations is of anxiety being the underlying driver resulting in an array of symptoms pursuing a solution to overwhelming anxiety. Children can experience anxiety in the following ways:

Mental processes or thoughts: worries about being hurt, either themselves or someone close to them; worries they will be laughed at.

Physically: increased heart rate, stomach ache, headache, vomiting, diarrhoea *(fight or flight response).*

Behaviour: fidgeting, pacing, crying, clingy and often some type of avoidance.

Typical anxiety disorders include:

Generalised anxiety disorder:

- Tendency to be worried or anxious about many areas of life;
- Unrealistic, excessive and persistent generalised anxiety about everyday situations, occurring most days;
- Accompanied by fatigue, restlessness, sleep disturbance;
- Leading to impairment in many areas of functioning.

Specific phobias:

- These can be common in childhood, different fears emerge at different ages;
- Fear described as a phobia when it is avoided persistently and daily function is impaired;
- Expressed by crying, tantrums, panic, freezing, clinging.

Social phobias:

- An exaggeration and persistence of the normal phase of stranger anxiety (normal up to 30 months, remember Mary Ainsworth's [1970] 'Strange Situation' discussed in Chapter 2);
- More than shyness, characterised by fear of humiliation or embarrassment;
- In the form of panic, freezing, withdrawal and autonomic arousal such as sweating, blushing, tremor, increased heart rate, some children are mute in certain situations;
- Poor prognosis if left untreated.

Separation anxiety disorders:

- Developmentally inappropriate persisting and excessive anxiety concerning separation;
- Often follows a stressful event such as an accident, bereavement or loss. In a domestic violence context a young person may not be prepared to leave the parental victim;
- Young children are more clingy, nightmares with themes of separation, sleeping alone;
- Age 9–12: severe distress on separation, withdrawn, somatic complaints;
- Adolescence: physical symptoms and somatisation features.

School phobia:

- More of a symptom than disorder often used with 'school refusal';
- Many reasons including separation anxiety, bullying, poor relationships, academic under-achievement.

Panic disorder:

- A fear or worry about having panic attacks;
- Recurrent unexpected attacks;
- Discrete episodes;
- Physical symptoms include: shortness of breath, palpitations, dizziness, chest pain, fear of losing control, etc.;
- More common in adolescence.

Post-traumatic stress disorder:

- A reaction to a serious traumatic event in which the child was extremely afraid or injured;
- Examples include physical, sexual abuse and or neglect events; events in the immediate and wider community such as local, national or global disasters;
- Normal to display some anxiety for a few weeks after the event, usually disappears, symptoms must be present for up to six months after the event;

- May keep having flashbacks and avoiding situations that remind them of the trauma;
- Jumpy, sleep difficulties and nightmares, intrusive images.

Obsessive compulsive disorder:

- Present when there are certain actions or thoughts that are repeated over and over again often for long periods;
- Can be quite complex and combined with tics and neurological problems and other extreme and unusual behaviours;
- Affected children will attempt to ignore, or suppress by 'performing compulsions' which are repetitive, purposeful behaviours often stereotypically;
- Parents often become caught up in complex rituals to avoid upset.

Activity

Anxiety case study: consider theoretical theories that can be applied.

Jean is 15 and was referred to CAMHS by her GP. She was seen by the consultant child and adolescent psychiatrist and diagnosed with school phobia/refusal. Jean was also diagnosed with clinical depression and commenced on anti-depressant medication and referred for some individual therapeutic work. The GP referred Jean to the incontinence service as she was unable to leave the house or travel far from home as she experienced urgency to pass urine. Jean was terrified of having an accident and not being able to get to a toilet on time. If she did venture out Jean would have worked out where the public toilets were on a shopping trip and how long car journeys would take, etc. She felt embarrassed by this which led to her avoiding going to friends' houses, not only from the point of view of the journey, but about having to ask to use the toilet at their homes. Jean was becoming more and more isolated and was tearful and distressed. She told a story of being attacked by some boys on a school trip a year ago. Police were called to the incident at the time. Jean's parents decided not to press charges and the matter was dropped.

There were other bullying incidents which took place at school and on journeys on the school bus. One serious incident concerned Jean being nearly strangled by another pupil on the school bus, using the seat belt. She managed to fight him off but did not tell her parents or anyone else about the incident.

Jean became more and more anxious about going to school and felt scared and unsafe.

Jean's parents were aware of the first assault but Jean did not tell them or anyone else about subsequent attacks. Both her parents tended to be accepting of whatever life 'dealt out' and tended not to challenge authority figures.

(Continued)

(Continued)

Social theory factors: school experiences, parenting style and stressful life events in terms of acute episodes and chronic bullying. School not deemed to be safe and understandably becoming a place to avoid, which seems a normal response.

Biological/medical theory: school phobia/refusal as defined by DSM 5 and ICD 10. Incontinence, problems with urinary retention. Depression similarly diagnosed and treatment including anti-depressant medication and talking therapies.

Psychological theory: Jean does have a capacity for safety seeking as she refuses to attend school, yet it has resulted in a clinical diagnosis.

SUICIDAL BEHAVIOUR AND DELIBERATE SELF-HARM

Historical note

It is worth reminding ourselves that until 1961 in the UK, suicide was illegal. Historically a suicide completer would not be buried in consecrated ground. In medieval times bodies would be buried at crossroads. The superstitious medieval population was fearful of death if the last rites had not been administered, which may mean the individual would be a potential threat to the living (Anderson, 1998). Interestingly a local paper reproduced two news items from 1852 and 1908 respectively, referring to suicide attempts. One item referred to a male who attempted 'self-destruction' by hanging. He was rescued by a neighbour when the man's wife raised the alarm. He was taken before the magistrate and admonished for the wickedness of his attempt and sent to prison for a week. The other article referred to a young woman of 23 before the city police court. She was charged with attempting to commit suicide by cutting her throat with a razor. Despite acknowledgement of her depression she was fined £10 together with an under-taking her husband looked after her (Grundy, 2008). These ideas remain around today with the tendency to describe a completed suicide as having been 'commit-ted', referring to the custodial sentence applied if one survived.

There continues to be ongoing stigma and shame and often negative attitudes towards suicide attempters in emergency room and accident and emergency set-tings (Mental Health Foundation, 2006; NSPCC, 2009). Later in the 20th century the phrase 'death trend' became adopted in the late 1950s and early 1960s where a study observed a large proportion of suicide attempters had experienced the loss of a significant figure, often tragically, prior to or during their own adolescent period. If self-destructive tendencies are a reaction to inner conflict, it may help to explain what links suicidal activity, becoming a chain reaction within populations, exam-ples of which exist throughout history (Moss and Hamilton, 1963 [1957], cited in Alvarez, 2002).

Considerations of risk and trigger factors tend to focus largely on external influences. The suicide cluster amongst young people in Bridgend, Wales, in 2008 established a link between internet sites and irresponsible media attention and was mooted as one of the reasons (Mickel, 2009). A similar view exists in the USA where recommendations for media responses have been developed to minimise the likelihood of copy-cat suicides. Similar proposals with regard to the media and internet are incorporated into the latest suicide strategy, Preventing Suicide in England (HM Government, 2012). Suicide clusters amongst young people are not new phenomena. Young people are often 'bonded' together, with the death of one compelling the death of another (Berman and Jobes, 1999 [1991]). Risk may also increase when young people identify with people who have taken their own life, whether they are a high-profile celebrity or another young person (Department of Health, 2011b).

The term 'suicidal behaviour' includes suicide and attempted suicide indicating an attempt to die with sufficient lethality (Berman and Jobes, 1999 [1991]). Deliberate self-harm includes, for example, poisoning, cutting, excessive alcohol, illegal drugs, hitting or burning oneself (Royal College of Psychiatrists, 2012a).

Adverse and abusive experiences in childhood are associated with an increased risk of suicide (Department of Health, 2011b). Looked after children are more at risk of experiencing mental health problems and they also potentially carry an increased risk of self-harming behaviours. Research by Hurry and Storey (1998, cited in NSPCC, 2009) showed that even though looked after children represent 1% of the population they represent 10% of children and young people presenting to accident and emergency departments following an act of deliberate self-harm.

Suicide attempts provide an active response to triggers acting as stressors. Suicide is often seen as a solution to intolerable overwhelming feelings rather than an explicit wish to die. The differences in self-harming behaviour, as opposed to deliberate self-harm or a suicide attempt are that with self-harm the person is in touch with their body through the physical reality of pain. Suicide attempts can be about a last sense of control over feelings of helplessness with the corresponding relief then experienced.

Consider the case of Shafilea Ahmed (Carter, 2012), whose parents were found guilty of murdering Shafilea in 2003. When on a visit to Pakistan Shafilea swallowed bleach, which would be regarded as attempted suicide. There was no evidence to suggest she was mentally ill but rather it was undoubtedly a response to overwhelming stressors and for her, seen as a solution to an intolerable situation. Interestingly and sadly in Shafilea's case the most pressing and immediate intervention would have been to ensure her safety from a child protection position.

The National Inquiry into Self-harm among Young People (Mental Health Foundation, 2006) suggests caution in viewing self-harm as a greater problem for young women. Young males engage in different sorts of self-harm such as hitting or breaking bones, which receives a different sort of attention and can sometimes be explained by an accident or a fight (Mental Health Foundation, 2006).

A survey of 6000 15- to 16-year-olds in England found that 6.9% engaged in self-harming behaviours with 12.6% of these presenting at a hospital for treatment. The survey found that self-harm is more common in females than males, at 11.2% and 3.2% respectively. Self-cutting accounted for 64% and self-poisoning for 30.7% as the main method used (Hawton et al., 2001). The majority of suicide attempters have already expressed their thoughts to others and 75% of completed suicides have had no contact with mental health services (Mental Health Foundation, 2006). According to the *National Service Framework for Children, Young People and Maternity Services* (Department of Health and Department for Education, 2004), 1985–95 saw an increase of 28.1% in teenage deliberate self-harm, which is often unidentified. Up to half were also likely to have a major depressive disorder and carry an increased risk of suicide. Suicide was noted as the most frequent cause of death amongst men and the third most frequent cause of death among women aged 15–24.

The suicide rate among young people continues to fall and is below that in the general population. However, young people are vulnerable to suicidal feelings. The risk is greater when they have mental health problems or behavioural disorder, misuse substances, have family breakdown or mental health problems or suicide in the family (Department of Health, 2011b).

The earlier Suicide Prevention Strategy for England (Department of Health, 2002) included various goals including a national collaboration for monitoring non-fatal deliberate self-harm and a pilot scheme targeting mental health promotion for young men. There was a proposal to reduce the availability and lethality of methods, with special reference to safer prescribing of anti-depressants and analgesics. There would be regular monitoring of suicides by age and gender (Department of Health, 2002). In the UK the most common form is poisoning (Royal College of Psychiatrists, 2012a).

In the same year the Royal College of Psychiatrists (2002) suggested a greater emphasis on prevention and earlier detection. Reductions in pack sizes of analgesics after 1998 led to a significant reduction in liver damage and completed suicides (Hawton et al., 2001). Analgesics including paracetamol are available as an over the counter medicine in pack sizes limited to 16 tablets per blister pack with additional limits on only being able to purchase two packs in a single transaction. If you consider, an overdose act takes a longer time period to accomplish if tablets have to be removed from blister packs and collected as opposed to swallowing a handful of tablets from an amount in a container. However seemingly minor, these are important considerations and offer restraint in suicidal acts with potential for a review and change of mind. Intent and motivation are key factors, which are mentioned below, and will be further discussed in Chapter 6.

The significance of high numbers of suicide attempts within the adolescent period no doubt has links with the developmental process. Adolescence is the most turbulent developmental period since infancy with the biggest challenges and changes in all three areas of biological, psychological and social change. Predisposing vulnerabilities can be activated during the adolescent phase (Anderson, 2008). Outside the adolescent period the only other time in life where such rapid changes, initiated by the hypothalamus, occur is in the womb (Waddell, 2002: 139).

Triggers influencing self-harm and suicidal behaviour include:

- Bullying
- Difficulties with parental and peer relationships
- Bereavement

- Earlier abusive experiences
- Difficulties with sexuality
- Problems with ethnicity, culture, religion
- Substance misuse and low self-esteem.

Contextual triggers include:

- Adverse family circumstances
- Dysfunctional relationships
- Domestic violence, poverty and parental criminality

- Time in local authority care
- Frequent punishments
- Family transitions.

All of the above become compounded by adolescent developmental pathology (Beautris, 1996, cited in Hider, 1998; Harrington, 2003). Bell (2000) describes that the cause given is actually the trigger precipitating suicidal behaviour. But it will often be the reason given by the young person, their families, and even doctors and other clinical staff. Reasons given might include an argument with a close friend or family member or failing exams. The notion of a trigger as an explanation often leads to a minimising of the level of seriousness surrounding the suicide attempt and is *never* about the stated reason. The reason identified is perhaps more of a rationalisation of the event rather than an explanation and it may be a frightening prospect for all concerned to even consider a serious mental disturbance. This is a very important point to bear in mind and is the key to understanding suicidal ideation. For example not all individuals who have arguments and fail exams make attempts on their lives, therefore those that do so for those reasons given are responding to a trigger (the argument, exam failure) to much deeper underlying intolerable problems. Suicide and suicidal ideation almost always take place within the context of relationships, which is the challenge to explore and understand. There is an emotional and psychological component. Exceptions are those responding to delusions or hallucinations linked to drug misuse or psychosis. Use of triggers as an explanation can lead to collusion and denial of the seriousness of the event, not only by family members but clinical staff also, and therefore it is highly risky in itself not to take the attempt seriously.

Deliberate self-harm including suicide attempts must be taken seriously and never minimised by describing somewhat trivial reasons such as relationship disagreements or exam failure. Those are triggers.

SELF-HARM

Self-harm and suicidal behaviour are emotional disorders on a similar continuum as both are in response to stress. A young person engaging in suicidal behaviour may wish to die or be ambivalent, whereas young people engaging in self-harming behaviour such as cutting do not necessarily have an active wish to die. Self-harm tends to be about coping whereas suicide is about giving up. It is worth noting that adolescents who self-harm carry a 100 times greater risk than that of the general population of completing a suicide in a subsequent year and that half of all completed suicides each year will have previously self-harmed (NICE, 2002). A research study of over 2000 pupils aged 15–16 years at secondary schools in Scotland showed that prevalence of self-harm was similar to England despite the suicide rate being twice as high. The report identified girls are three times more likely to report self-harm than boys. The most common motive described was to get relief from 'a terrible state of mind'. Almost 4 in 10 teenagers in the study reported they wanted to die (O'Connor et al., 2009). Self-harm is a major public health issue with estimates that as many as one in 15 young people self-harm in the UK, higher than the rest of Europe. There is universal misunderstanding about self-harm by the people closest to them often leading to poor responses (Mental Health Foundation, 2006). Self-harm continues to be stigmatised, often remaining hidden, which can lead to guilt and shame often compounded by the reactions of others (NSPCC, 2009). The differences in self-harming behaviour, as opposed to an intention to kill oneself, are that with self-harm the person is in touch with his/her body through the physical reality of pain. When the wish for self-preservation against physical danger is lacking, as in a suicide attempt, leading to an attack on the body, it is in part about taking control over feelings of helplessness with the corresponding relief thereby then experienced.

As will be discussed in Chapter 2, infantile experiences are internalised and attachment patterns laid down, affecting later relationships. Events that trigger self-harming behaviour are actions rooted in old patterns and wounds. However these are not necessarily about trauma as not all who self-harm have been victims of abuse or trauma in childhood. The skin becomes a medium for communication (Gardner, 2001). Consider other powerful body modification similarities where the skin becomes a medium of communication through decoration with tattooing and piercing. Where reasons motivating modifications to the external 'skin' or surface may be found 'under the skin', within the internal world (Lemma, 2010: 2). Physical pain is often easier to manage than emotional pain, and when inflicted can change mood which in turn can be habit forming. Cutting releases endorphins into the system providing a brief calming effect combined with serotonin as a mood enhancer and therefore experienced as a form of relief. There is also something about first aid 'patching up' and 'repairing' either by the individual or helpers, with these repairing acts experienced as therapeutic. Very often the shocking quality communicates the rawness of emotions and impulses and is an essential aspect of the behaviour (Turp, 1999, cited in Gardner, 2001: 8).

Activity

Have a look at the following case study. Consider Jim in relation to the risk and resilience model discussed earlier in the chapter. Similarly think about the theoretical models in relation to the information about Jim.

Jim is 14 and was referred to Tier 3 CAMHS by his GP for assessment. Jim was self-harming by burning his finger tips. There were concerns over suicidal ideation and possible clinical depression.

Jim lives with his mother, younger brother and stepfather. His brother has a significant physical illness requiring a lot of medical interventions and hos-pitalisations. As a child Jim's mum had been bullied by an overbearing father.

Jim's father lives with his third wife. Jim's father was in care as a child. Jim and his brother visit them once a week and sometimes stay over. Jim would like to spend more time with dad but dad is very rigid around routines and the times they spend and stay with each other. There was a recent incident where Jim ran away from home and dad wondered if Jim should go into care.

Jim has a passion for music, both writing and playing the guitar. Therefore burn-ing his finger tips is significant for Jim and also very punishing.

Jim feels guilty, thinking he is the only 'well' member of the household, stating his one wish for his brother was not to be ill, feeling they could all be happy again then.

There have been reported incidents from school of Jim being bullied. He often becomes over-involved in sorting out other friends' problems. There is a real sense of him trying to repair others in the absence of being able to repair his family.

Risk and resilience factors for Jim

For Jim the risk factors mainly sit in his family and contextual and systemic factors: parental conflict, family breakdown, rejecting relationships (dad), potential bereavement issues regarding Jim's brother (loss of potential for normal health), significant life events, whether dad has been able to adapt to Jim's changing developmental needs. An evident potential resilience factor is his musical talents. Jim's mum is trying to get help for him.

Jim: theoretical interpretations

Jim's presentation will be interpreted as illness (medical theory) and he is likely to have a diagnosis of clinical depression, he may also have been traumatised through bullying and family breakdown experiences. There is limited information regarding psychologi-cal theories but we can be curious about attachment perhaps given both Jim's parents experiences. Jim feels a responsibility to be 'well' and feels responsible for 'repair'. He seeks to repair others (peers) in the absence of repairs in his family. Social, systematic and environmental theories are strongly evident in this case and probably represent the most significant model. There is the context of Jim's family: illness, family breakdown, relationship patterns and stressful life events. Parental experiences and generational issues cannot be ignored either. Mum has an experience of bullying in her childhood. Dad has been in care. Both parents bring to their own family, becoming parents them-selves, their own 'ghosts from the nursery' or early experiences. Jim's father is only par-tially available for Jim with an imminent sense of unavailability present.

EATING DISORDERS

Terminology

Eating disorders comprise a collection of disorders including anorexia nervosa, bulimia nervosa and binge eating disorder in DSM 5; in ICD 10 similarly and also atypical eating disorders and eating disorder, unspecified.

Prognosis

Sixty per cent of individuals treated for anorexia nervosa will have a good outcome, 30% will have an intermediate outcome and 10% will have a poor outcome (Bryant-Waugh, 2003). There are similar statistics for both adults and young people. The average duration of illness is five years. It has a mortality rate which is twice the level of any other illness and the highest death rate of my mental illness (Treasure and Alexander, 2013). It is extremely serious and can be persistently difficult to treat, requiring specialist interventions which at times also may include sectioning under the Mental Health Act 2007. There is no lower age limit for the use of compulsory powers under the Act. The Mental Capacity Act 2005 applies to over-16s. Young people with anorexia nervosa have the highest bed occupancy in Tier 4 in-patient CAMHS and for the longest periods of time. The average in-patient stay is 12 months, so there are obvious implications not only in terms of resources but the psychological and sociological components and impact for both the young person and his/her family. In-patient units are a specialised centralised regional provision around the country so often young people requiring admission find themselves a long way from home. Even with successful treatment and recovery, patients can be left with long-term problems of physical health including osteoporosis, infertility and depression (Nunn, 2013). It must be remembered re-feeding in a specialist unit or hospital to a healthy weight is only a relatively minor aspect of what is long-term treatment.

Prevalence

The most frequent age of onset is between 15 and 35 years and approximately 0.3–0.5% of the population up to 18 develops anorexia nervosa. Figures for bulimia are 1% although bulimia is rare under 12 with an average onset of 15–18 years compared to 15 years for anorexia. Gender ratio is female to male 4:1 for under 12 years and 9:1 for the age range 13–18 years. Anorexia nervosa is not a disease of the middle classes as is sometimes thought and crosses all cultural and social backgrounds. There is increasing global recognition especially in countries experiencing economic change alongside the changing roles of women in these countries (Cullen, 2011). It is interesting to note that in the parts of the world where food is in short supply eating disorders are virtually unknown (Lawrence, 2008).

Diagnosis

Diagnostic criteria for anorexia nervosa according to ICD 10 includes a body weight maintained at least 15% below that expected or a BMI (body mass index) of 17.5 or less. BMI is calculated differently for children and young people as compared to adults. There must be self-induced weight loss by avoidance of fattening foods and at least one of the following: self-induced vomiting, self-induced purging, excessive exercise, use of appetite suppressants and/or diuretics. Diagnostic criteria also include body image distortion in females and absence of more than three menstrual cycles (Treasure and Karwautz, 2004). In DSM 5 (American Psychiatric Association, 2013) the requirement for amenorrhoea has been eliminated (previously included in DSM IV). Individuals are required to be at a significantly low body weight for their developmental stage. If the onset of anorexia nervosa is pre-pubertal puberty becomes delayed or arrested.

Diagnostic criteria for bulimia include: persistent preoccupation with eating and an irresistible craving for food often consuming vast amounts in a short space of time. The patient tries to counteract the fattening effects by self-induced vomiting, purgative abuse, alternating periods of starvation or use of drugs as appetite suppressants or diuretics. There will be a morbid dread of fatness and often a previous history of anorexia nervosa. The similarities between anorexia nervosa and bulimia are diets, food rules, binges and intense exercising.

Theoretical models and anorexia nervosa

It is generally considered, as with other mental health disorders, that eating disorders arise from a combination of theoretical models, namely biological, psychological and social, systemic and environmental factors. These will be demonstrated below with a case study.

Genetic vulnerability has been identified, with female relatives of sufferers of anorexia being 11.4 times as likely to suffer as the control group and 3.7 times more likely for bulimia (Strober et al., 1999). More recent research also suggests a strong genetic link and predisposition, with neuro-imaging showing differences in brain structure in anorexia nervosa patients. This would suggest anorexia nervosa is a disease combination of both biological and psychological features. The research demonstrates that anorexia nervosa is not a lifestyle choice but rather an inherent gene which is most probably present and becomes vulnerable when exposed to other factors (Lask et al., 2012). Again this new research underpins the nature versus nurture discussion, in that development and mental health and ill health take place within a contextual combination of inherent characteristics and it is about how these articulate with the environment and experiences. This rather undermines an argument often presented that western societal values and media representations of thin role models and association with positive attributes of attractiveness and popularity predict development of eating disorders (Stice, 2002). Anorexia has previously been referred to as the 'slimmer's disease'. Dieting in itself does not cause anorexia, although many who do go on to develop anorexia will have started out by dieting which then seems to act as a trigger for some individuals.

There are undoubtedly certain high-risk groups. Vulnerable individuals are not helped by internet websites promoting anorexia, especially amongst those groups working in areas which emphasise a fit or thin body such as sport and fashion (Lawrence, 2008). With perfectionism implicated as both a risk and a maintaining factor (Fairburn and Harrison, 2003) activities such as sport and fashion may well appeal to those with perfectionist traits, something which McDougall (1989) referred to as the 'theatre of the body'.

Other predisposing factors centre on the negotiation of transitional points, for example the negotiation of adolescence in combination with an adverse life event such as bereavement, parental divorce and sexual abuse, together with a psychological vulnerability. There are also similarities with self-harm and suicidal behaviour in that there will always is a contextual background of either relationship or attachment difficulties, even if they are not immediately apparent. Anorexia nervosa could also be regarded as self-harming behaviour, which it is and it must be also remembered that sadly it also takes some young people and adults ultimately to their deaths.

There are similarities with the 'triggers' described in relation to suicide attempts and the 'trigger' being the reason often given. So the media and societal attitudes towards thinness often cited as '*reasons*' are not reasons in themselves but rather act as contributing factors or triggers. These are social theory factors and they would not operate in isolation of psychological and biological theories but rather as a combination of contributing factors from all domains. The interaction of these models is unique to each individual in terms of their life story and circumstances. The task is to understand this articulation, which will be discussed in more detail in Chapter 6 and is demonstrated here by the following case study.

Activity

Consider the application of theoretical models to the following case study:

Jane is 13 and has been admitted to a Tier 4 child and adolescent in-patient unit, following a diagnosis of anorexia nervosa. On admission she had a BMI of 11.9 and had not yet commenced menstruation. Prior to this there had been a two-year history of restricted eating and weight loss. As a child Jane had attended ballet and dance classes, and she would recall her dance teacher saying she was too fat to be a ballet dancer; Jane was 8 at the time. Jane began to restrict her food intake when she was 11 and this coincided with her transition to secondary school. Unfortunately Jane was not able to go to her choice of school. Both of Jane's parents are working in professional occupations and Jane has two younger siblings.

Jane has a distorted body image, has perfectionist traits, does not believe she is 'good enough' and finds criticism difficult to deal with. Jane does not seem to 'act out' in any traditional 'teenagey' ways. She does not easily express how she feels and tends to keep everything to herself.

During her in-patient stay Jane was diagnosed with depression and prescribed anti-depressant medication. Jane remained in hospital for a year and was discharged to her local Tier 3 CAMHS team.

Medical/biological theory: Jane has been diagnosed with anorexia nervosa. There may well be a genetic component if there were other family members with anorexia, perhaps from previous generations.

Psychological theory: Jane may find negotiating a transition point difficult when moving to secondary school and combined with emerging adolescence. This is also seen in her not appearing to be very 'teenagey'. In addition, Jane has perfectionist traits and low self-esteem, tending to internalise rather than externalise feelings.

Social and environmental theories: Factors such as Jane's dance teacher telling her she was too fat may have acted as a trigger leading to development of AN when combined with other psychological factors as above.

EARLY ONSET PSYCHOSIS

Psychosis describes an individual as being out of touch with reality and is a collection of signs and symptoms describing a particular mental state (Dogra et al., 2009). Psychotic illness is serious and can affect all age groups although a first episode/early onset psychosis typically occurs in young adulthood. The peak age of onset is 15–19 in both males and females and there is controversy about prevalence in pre-pubertal children, accepted rates are much higher after puberty. Early onset is rare, but 60% of adult cases reported to have childhood onset (James, 2003: 121). The national average annual incidence is about 15 per 100,000 (Vostanis, 2007). Early onset psychosis is relatively rare but nevertheless very serious. Current diagnostic criteria only applies to adults, so there are limitations when applying to young people (NICE, 2006). A single episode of psychosis does not necessarily preclude schizophrenia or an affective disorder. Anyone experiencing a psychotic episode needs urgent assessment, risk assessment and treatment (Dogra et al., 2009). There are high rates of completed suicides and 20% of sufferers make a significant suicide attempt within a five-year period following diagnosis (Strober et al., 1999).

There are two forms of psychotic illness: schizophrenia and bipolar affective disorder (formerly known as manic depressive disorder). Schizophrenia is the most common form of psychosis. It is a serious mental disorder affecting thinking, emotions and behaviour. There is however a view that a diagnostic term such as schizophrenia is unhelpful and unreliable given the changing range of problems coming under one umbrella term. Not only that, there are significant stigmatising problems for sufferers (Gaughan, 2011). Symptoms of schizophrenia are described as either 'positive', '*added to the person*', or 'negative', '*taken away from the person*', and sufferers usually experience a combination. 'Positive' symptoms include delusions, thought disorder and hallucinations. 'Negative' symptoms include being withdrawn, a loss of interest, poor hygiene, isolation and problems with concentration. The main features of bipolar affective disorder are extreme mood changes.

Risk factors for psychotic illness include a family history, with stress or extreme life events acting as a trigger factor. Schizophrenia has an increased risk if there is a diagnosis of a close relative such as a parent or sibling. In young people common triggers of psychosis include substance misuse, medical reasons such as fever or epilepsy, or side effects from prescribed medication (Dogra et al., 2009). Substance misuse includes particularly cannabis, LSD, ecstasy and speed (Royal College of Psychiatrists, 2012b, 2012c).

Trauma can significantly impact on development. Schreier et al. (2009, cited in Gaughan, 2011) found that the risk for psychosis was doubled if bullying was persistent and long-standing, which is in line with the risk and resilience model discussed earlier in the chapter. Whitfield et al. (2005, cited in Gaughan, 2011) found a significant connection between childhood trauma and hallucinations. In both schizophrenia and bipolar disorder there are abnormalities in brain chemistry. There is no single cause but rather a probability of multiple gene factors (*biological model*) articulating with environmental factors (*social environmental model/ theory*) which then leads to psychosis.

It is a common feature to have other co-morbidities: 70% of hospitalised adolescents with bipolar disorder have a diagnosis of ADHD; 39% have substance abuse and dependence; 30% suffer with anxiety disorders and may have been previously diagnosed with schizophrenia (Strober et al., 1999).

Zubin and Spring's (1977) 'Stress Vulnerability Model', despite its age, usefully demonstrates how we are all vulnerable to psychosis, but some are more vulnerable than others. An individual's vulnerability is the *disposition* of the person to manifest symptoms of serious mental illness.

> *Inborn* vulnerability: genetically determined, reflected in the neurophysiology of the organism (biological/medical).
>
> *Acquired* vulnerability: specific to individual life experience; can include specific disease, perinatal complications, family experience, adolescent peer interactions, previous life events (psychological and social environmental).

So as we will discuss in Chapter 2, potential innate vulnerability such as inherent temperament, genetic predisposition and how these articulate with social and environmental factors and how these are experienced are all contributing factors.

SUBSTANCE MISUSE

Substance misuse is a broad term encompassing the harmful use of any psychotropic substance, including alcohol and either legal or illicit drugs. Such use is usually, but not always, regarded as a problem if there is evidence of dependence. Forty per cent of people with psychosis misuse substances at some point in their lifetime, at least double the rate seen in the general population (NICE, 2011). It is also worth remembering that emerging personality disorders do so from a context often of self-harm, depression, eating disorders and substance misuse. Diagnosis is unlikely to take place until adulthood due to the complexity of adolescent pathology. There is also stigma attached to '*labelling*' anyone at an early age, given the implications (Mind, 2012; NICE, 2009).

Young people experience a wide range and diversity of substance misuse with multiple effects and wider societal implications. Adult services tend to focus on dependence and management whereas young people's services have a focus on harm reduction with concerns on developmental processes. Single episodes can have serious life-threatening outcomes (Brodie and Reed, 2011; Crome, 2004, cited in Brodie and Reed, 2011). Regular substance misuse leads to serious disruption in education, relationships and long-term physical and emotional health. Most adult substance misuse and dependence begin in early adolescence. Adult mental health problems and social disruption are linked to early onset substance misuse.

Young people are less likely than adults to present at services with substance misuse problems. Substance use can also be thought of as a normal part of adolescent risk taking behaviour. Brodie and Reed (2011: 241) have some useful definitions.

The following indicate areas of vulnerability to developing a substance abuse problem:

- Parental substance misuse and parental mental health problems.
- Pregnant drug users are at increased risk of postnatal mental health problems, affecting attachment.
- Demands of substance dependence with an infant with neonatal abstinence syndrome can negatively affect formation of secure attachment.
- Children raised in substance misusing households believe exposures to high-risk situations are normal.
- Concentrated in areas of high social deprivation, inadequate housing, poverty and low employment.
- Substance misuse does not exist as an independent problem but rather as part of a cluster of other difficulties which must be addressed.

Activity

Have a look at the following case study and consider where the areas of vulnerability are using the theoretical models:

Tyler is 17 and has been experiencing unusual ideas and experiences for about 18 months, alongside deterioration in his daily functioning and an increase in his cannabis use. He dropped out of school before completing his exams.

His mother became increasingly concerned about his state of mind over the past year and about three months ago finally convinced him to visit his GP; who referred him on to the local CAMHS Tier 3 team; who in turn passed his case to a local Early Intervention in Psychosis Service. They have just completed an assessment with him.

Tyler is presenting with paranoid and anxious thoughts about other young people in his community, some of whom he believed had also harassed and bullied him during school. He believes that people are out to get him, though reports from his mother suggest there isn't anyone in particular that has a problem with him but

(Continued)

(Continued)

this increasingly strange behaviour has led to people making comments. He has reported some intermittent hearing of a voice that tends to criticise him. Tyler has experienced low mood and has had some suicidal thoughts on occasions but says he wouldn't act upon these. On the whole, though, he feels numb to feelings other than anxiety. He is quite socially isolated but is a member of a darts team that he goes to with his father sometimes.

Tyler's family and developmental history

Tyler's parents divorced 10 years ago. He is of dual heritage with his mother being Sri Lankan and his father being white British. He has an older brother of 30, Jason, with a diagnosis of schizophrenia. Jason was in a psychiatric hospital during his twenties. Family life had been frequently stressful and often orientated around Jason's needs and intermittent involvement with the family.

Soon after his 16th birthday Tyler's relationship with his mother deteriorated following high levels of conflict and he was thrown out, leading to an independent living flat in his neighbourhood – a relatively deprived area of an otherwise largely affluent town. Tyler experienced what he describes as persistent bullying in school and feels this continues in his locality. Some of this has related to people's knowledge of Jason. He had some friendships during school but hasn't maintained these relationships. He briefly hung around with a group of young people but was worried about increasing police attention they were receiving and now does not see them in a friendship capacity.

Inborn vulnerability: Tyler may have a genetic predisposition to developing psychosis as there is a close family member with a diagnosis (his brother) (biological/medical).

Acquired vulnerability: Tyler is also at risk here due to traumatic life events such as bullying, parental discord and family breakdown (social and environmental factors).

Tyler is exhibiting concerning signs of potential psychosis coinciding and combined with an increased use of cannabis. The two may be interrelated, meaning psychotic symptoms may be as a result of cannabis use or they may have emerged without substance misuse as he has a close family member with a diagnosis.

NEURO-DEVELOPMENTAL CONDITIONS

Neuro-developmental conditions include a large group of 'disorders' commencing in early life and persisting into adulthood. There can be some confusion with the term 'learning difficulties', which is also seen in service provision with an overlap of children and young people with neuro-developmental conditions presenting in either CAMHS tiers, community paediatric or learning disability services. Terminology fluctuates between conditions, disorders and difficulties and is interchangeable. Within the context of the chapter the focus will be on attention deficit hyperactivity disorder

(ADHD) (sometimes referred to as hyperkinetic disorder), conduct disorder (CD) and autistic spectrum conditions (ASC), as these are the most frequent and more common conditions you are likely to come across. Although it should be noted there are several other classifications including pervasive developmental disorder, pervasive oppositional defiant disorder, attention deficit disorder, dyslexia and so on.

ATTENTION DEFICIT HYPERACTIVITY DISORDER

ADHD can best be understood as a neurological difficulty which interferes with an individual's availability for learning (Silver, 1990).

> More recently, extensive biological investigations of both ADHD and hyperkinetic disorder have yielded some neuroimaging and molecular genetic associations; neurocognitive theories have emerged; and there is a better understanding of the natural history and the risks that hyperactive behaviour imposes. Nevertheless, the disorder remains one that is defined at a behavioural level, and its presence does not imply a neurological disease. (National Collaborating Centre for Mental Health, 2009:15)

There is a case study (Joe) in Chapter 2 which demonstrates this potential. Characteristics of ADHD include a triad or constellation of impairments in the following three areas:

- Poor concentration
- Hyperactivity
- Impulsiveness.

It is important to recognise that displaying the above behaviours does not necessarily mean ADHD is the explanation. These behaviours may indicate psychological causes. Think about how you might behave if you were in a stressful situation, experiencing stress and anxiety; all of the above areas are likely to show changes. A key factor is the persistence and frequency in all domains.

A problem for children and young people is that their ADHD impairments can impact significantly on educational experiences and attainment. Young people with ADHD have a higher rate of behavioural and disruptive disorders and as we have already seen earlier in this chapter they are disproportionately represented in the youth justice service. Children with ADHD often fail to regulate activity and they are less able to evaluate their responses beforehand or subsequently. Exhortations to 'try harder' or 'learn to concentrate' are impossible to fulfil and these are often made repeatedly by those who teach and look after them.

The range of possible lifetime impairment extends to educational and occupational underachievement, dangerous driving, difficulties in carrying out daily activities such as shopping and organising household tasks, in making and keeping friends, in intimate relationships (for example, excessive disagreement) and with child care (NICE, 2008: 5).

As with other disorders ADHD is classified in both ICD 10 (hyperkinetic disorder) and in DSM 5. Severe ADHD corresponds approximately to the ICD 10 diagnosis of hyperkinetic disorder. This is defined as when hyperactivity, impulsivity and inattention are all present in multiple settings, and when impairment affects multiple domains in multiple settings. Part of the assessment process would include collecting information from parents and from educational settings. Diagnosis is a matter of clinical judgement which considers the severity of impairment, pervasiveness, individual factors and familial and social context (NICE, 2008).

There are strong genetic influences and often history taking reveals other family members exhibiting ADHD traits that are undiagnosed; this is significantly so in earlier generations where ADHD was unrecognised. No single gene has yet been identified.

Environmental factors include maternal drug and alcohol use in pregnancy. In addition, ongoing effects of individual and parental substance misuse and poor or hostile parenting also need to be considered. In the UK, a survey of 10,438 children between the ages of 5 and 15 years found that 3.62% of boys and 0.85% of girls had ADHD (Ford et al., 2003, cited in National Collaborating Centre for Mental Health, 2009: 26). ADHD seems to be approximately four times more common in boys than girls. Globally there are variations of between 1 and 20% which may be explained by cultural differences and how symptoms are measured. Overall a figure of 5% is thought to be more accurate (Jones and Claveirole, 2011).

It is thought that diagnostic and treatment criteria are influenced by social and cultural factors. In the USA ADHD has been long recognised and treated more robustly than in other parts of the world. This may well be a reflection of a strong diagnostic medical model which interprets and classifies behaviours. In Britain there can be a reluctance to diagnose children and resistance to treatment interventions as these usually include medication. Parents and young people can be understandably concerned about this.

Psychological factors include severe early psychosocial deprivation such as experienced in poor institutional care. ADHD is more prevalent in families where there are disruptive relationships (National Collaborating Centre for Mental Health, 2009: 29). You can see there is correlation between all theoretical domains. Risk factors do not occur in isolation, nor can they be explained by a single theory but rather it is about the interaction and articulation between all domains.

A pharmacological approach is recommended as first line treatment (in conjunction with parenting and individual programmes) for ADHD using a prescribed psychostimulant (methylphenidate) (NICE, 2008). Medication can help children with concentration so has a valid use in supporting children in school settings. Young people I have known have been successfully treated with methylphenidate and tell me it buys them *thinking time* so impulsivity is reduced and that it does help significantly with concentration. It can help with symptom (triad of impairments) control, and does not remain in the system for more than a few hours. Treatment 'holidays' can be taken so for example the young person may not wish to take medication at the weekend or in the school holidays. There are however side effects including loss of appetite and difficulty getting to sleep. Children and young people need close medical monitoring as there are implications in terms of physical development if appetite and subsequently diet is suppressed.

A multifaceted and multi-agency approach in the management of ADHD includes parent and teacher training in behavioural techniques as well as individual support for the young person. It can be helpful to reframe the negative symptoms of ADHD in terms of positive aspects. It is not always helpful to focus on reducing 'unwanted' behaviours, alternatively it is better to harness the positives (remember the resilience model and having a skill or talent). There is potential for these young people as they usually have energy and enthusiasm by the bucket load. They have a 'feet first' activist approach which during childhood and adolescence can get them into trouble but needs to be seen as also having advantages. But it can be difficult to 'fit into systems' especially the demands of education, which can be stacked against a child or young person with ADHD.

CONDUCT DISORDERS

Conduct disorders, and associated antisocial behaviour, are the most common mental and behavioural problems in children and young people. The Office of National Statistics (ONS) surveys of 1999 and 2004 reported that their prevalence was 5% among children and young people aged between 5 and 16 years. Conduct disorders nearly always have a significant impact on functioning and quality of life. The 1999 ONS survey demonstrated that conduct disorders have a steep social class gradient, with a three to fourfold increase in prevalence in social classes D and E compared with social class A. The 2004 survey found that almost 40% of looked-after children, those who had been abused and those on child protection or safeguarding registers had a conduct disorder. (NICE, 2013: 4)

Conduct disorder refers to aggressive, destructive and disruptive behaviours in childhood that are serious and likely to impair a child's development. In DSM 5 there is a distinction between oppositional defiant disorder (characterised by recurrent negativistic defiant, disobedient and hostile behaviours) and conduct disorder which includes a presence of repetitive persistent violations of societal norms and other people's basic rights. In ICD 10 oppositional and conduct problems are both included under the heading of conduct disorder. Many behaviours included in the diagnosis are common in normal child development, but when they are persistent and frequent they bring increased risks in later life including: antisocial behaviours, a range of psychiatric disorders, educational and work failure and relationship difficulties (Moffitt et al., 2002). Conduct disorder is more common in boys than girls (NICE, 2013). There is frequently co-morbidity with other illness including substance misuse, anxiety and ADHD. It is considered there is substantial heritability but little is known about the mechanisms. Children with conduct disorder are likely to have: lower IQ, poor verbal skills, low tolerance of frustration, lack of anxious inhibition or rule breaking, problems of hyperactivity and executive function, impaired attention and concentration (Henry et al., 1996). Individual risk factors include low school achievement and impulsiveness; family risk factors include parental contact with the criminal justice system and child abuse; social risk factors include low family income and little education (NICE, 2013). Parenting practices in families of conduct-disordered children are reported as often hostile, critical, with harsh discipline, a lack of consistent rules, low monitoring of behaviours and parental disagreements.

A child or young person presenting with conduct disorder is doing so in a context of all of the theoretical domains. Where there is a combination of inherited vulnerability plus negative parenting, especially early negative affect and intrusive control these factors contribute to the development and persistence of conduct problems. These are often highly vulnerable young people and can be a risk to themselves and others. There is a discussion in Chapter 3 about the Edlington case of two brothers who both had a diagnosis of conduct disorder. Lord Carlile in his review noted a lack of robustness in agencies working together (Carlile, 2012). NICE (2013) guidelines now recommend a combination of person-centred care. For example, parent training and other multi-modal interventions such as family therapy and methylphenidate for management of the ADHD aspects.

AUTISTIC SPECTRUM CONDITIONS

Autistic spectrum conditions or disorders form a very broad variation in presentation. 'Spectrum' indicates that while sharing the same condition there is a wide range of difficulties experienced in different ways. On a scale of 0–100 on the spectrum and starting at zero, a social and communicative person would appear. Moving further along the spectrum someone with a few autistic traits such as a need for routine would appear. The stronger the autistic traits the further along the spectrum, so at 100 there would be a person with no speech and limited responses to others (Muggleton, 2012: 31). There may be accompanying learning disabilities. It is a lifelong condition and unlike all the other conditions discussed in this chapter has a biological origin and is a disorder of development. Autistic people often experience sensitivity to sounds, touch, tastes, smells, light or colours (National Autistic Society, 2013).

Autism is characterised by a triad of features related to functioning in all situations:

- Impairment of social communication
- Impairment of social understanding
- Impairment in social imagination and play.

There are also accompanying and ritualistic stereotyped interests and behaviours. These are usually evident from infancy although they may not be recognised at that point. Play is often a preoccupation with repetitive activities. I recall meeting a referred boy age 7 for an assessment in Tier 2 CAMHS. He had been referred by a paediatrician over concerns about aggressive behaviour (he had kicked the dinner ladies at school). The boy had very sadly lost his mother who died after a long fight with cancer. Understandably it was thought his behaviour may have been a response to that and that he would benefit from some help. However when my colleague and I first met with him and his dad it was very clear quite quickly to us that he was demonstrating some autistic traits. There were lots of toys in the room but he spent the whole time taking apart and putting together a transformer toy. He did some drawing at one point but these were of train engines. Dad said that was the only thing he would draw and he only played with a transformer toy at home. He did not really interact with us in a conversational way and only in monosyllabic answers. He also spoke in an American accent. We referred him on to the learning disabilities service for children where he was assessed and diagnosed as on the autistic spectrum. The problem had been that the dinner ladies and other school staff were, as an act of kindness, giving him a hug. He could not bear the physical touch and as an autistic characteristic was sensitive to touch. To get away from them he would lash out. Quite a long time later he was still speaking in an American accent. Having a diagnosis does not in itself change anything but it can help parents and teachers to understand a child's needs and put in place supportive measures.

Autism in Britain was first labelled as childhood psychosis at the beginning of the 20th century. In 1944 it was named 'Kanner's syndrome', and then in the latter part of the 20th century 'autism' (Wing, 1996). Asperger's syndrome was identified in 1944 although it took until 1979 for Asperger's work to be translated from German to English. It wasn't until 1991 that the term Asperger's syndrome was recognised in Britain. The difference between autism and Asperger's syndrome is that 'Aspies' are of average or higher intelligence and develop language skills in the normal developmental way, while the reverse is true for autistic people (Bradshaw, 2013: 55).

Again as with children and young people with ADHD it is helpful to consider positives for Asperger's children. Although it has to be acknowledged they are often the victims of bullying and misunderstanding. Their strengths can be in individual sports for example. Another trait is honesty; never ask *'does my bum look big in this?'* If you are not prepared for an honest response, do not ask if the truth is going to hurt! Similarly language needs to be straightforward, if you ask an 'Aspie' to 'hold your horses', i.e. slow down, you will have a puzzled response, wondering – where exactly are the horses?

CONCLUSION

As we have seen child and adolescent mental health covers many areas, some of which have only been touched upon in the chapter. Children and young people are at significant risk of developing mental health problems within the context of a developing individual. This is certainly the case for particularly vulnerable children such as looked after children. CAMHS and accompanying interventions provide a window of opportunity to address problems before these proceed into adulthood, where they will be much more resistant, complex and harder to deal with. In keeping with Winnicott's quote, '*there is no such thing as an infant ... show me someone caring for the baby*', children and young people presenting with difficulties are always thought of systemically and contextually which is where the clues will lie if we are able to find them. Always be curious.

REFERENCES

Ainsworth, M. (1970) Attachment, Exploration, and Separation: Illustrated by the Behavior of One-year-olds in a Strange Situation. *Child Development*, 41 (1): 49–67.

Alvarez, A. (2002) *The Savage God: A Study of Suicide*. London: Bloomsbury.

American Psychiatric Association (2013) *Diagnostic and Statistical Manual of Mental Disorders*, 5th edn. Arlington, DC: American Psychiatric Association. Available from: www.psychiatry.org/dsm5 (accessed July 2013).

Anderson, R. (1998) *Facing it Out: Clinical Perspectives on Adolescent Disturbance*. London: Karnac.

Anderson, R. (2008) A Psychoanalytic Approach to Suicide in Adolescents. In Briggs, S., Lemma, A. and Crouch, W. (eds) *Relating to Self-Harm and Suicide: Psychoanalytic Perspectives on Practice, Theory and Prevention*. Hove: Routledge, pp. 61–71.

Barber, P., Brown, R. and Martin, D. (2012) *MH Law in England and Wales: A Guide for Mental Health Professionals*. London: Sage.

Bell, D. (2000) Who is Killing What or Whom? Some Notes on the Internal Phenomenology of Suicide. *Psychoanalytic Psychotherapy*, 15 (1): 21–37.

Berman, A. and Jobes, D. (1999 [1991]) *Adolescent Suicide Assessment and Intervention*. Washington, DC: American Psychological Association.

Bowlby, J. (2008 [1988]) *A Secure Base*. London: Routledge.

Bradshaw, S. (2013) *Asperger's Syndrome – That Explains Everything: Strategies for Education, Life and Just About Everything Else*. London: Jessica Kingsley.

British Medical Association Board of Science (2006) *Child and Adolescent Mental Health: A Guide for Healthcare Professionals*. London: BMA.

Brodie, L. and Reed, J. (2011) Misuse of Substances. In Claveirole, A. and Gaughan, M. (eds) *Understanding Children and Young People's Mental Health*. Chichester: Wiley-Blackwell, pp. 239–55.

Bryant-Waugh, R. (2003) Eating Disorders. In Skuse, D. *Child Psychology and Psychiatry: An Introduction*. Oxford: The Medicine Publishing Company.

Carlile, Lord (2012) *The Edlington Case: A Review by Lord Carlile of Berriew CBE QC at the Request of The Rt Hon Michael Gove MP Secretary of State for Education*. Available from: www.gov.uk/government/uploads/system/uploads/attachment_data/file/177098/The_Edlington_case.pdf (accessed August 2013).

Carter, H. (2012) Shafilea Ahmed's Parents Jailed for her Murder. *The Guardian*. Available from: www.guardian.co.uk/uk/2012/aug/03/shafilea-ahmed-parents-guilty-murder (accessed August 2012).

Chimat (Child and Maternal Health Observatory) (2012) *Targeted Mental Health in Schools (TaMHS)*. Available from: www.chimat.org.uk/camhs/schools/tamhs (accessed August 2012).

Coleman, F. and Hagell, A. (eds) (2007) *Adolescence Risk and Resilience Against the Odds*. Chichester: John Wiley.

Cullen, G. (2011) Eating Disorders. In Claveirole, A. and Gaughan, M. (eds) *Understanding Children and Young People's Mental Health*. Chichester: Wiley-Blackwell, pp. 149–64.

Department for Education (2013) *Children Looked after in England (including Adoption and Care Leavers) Year Ending 31 March 2012*. Available from: www.gov.uk/government/uploads/system/uploads/attachment_data/file/219210/sfr20-2012v2.pdf (accessed July 2013).

Department of Health (2002) *Suicide Prevention Strategy for England. Executive Summary*. Available from: www.dh.gov.uk/en/Publicationsandstatistics/Publications/PublicationsPolicyAndGuidance/DH_4009474 (accessed August 2012).

Department of Health (2007) *Teenage Parents Next Steps: Guidance for Local Authorities and PCT's*. Available from: www.changeforchildren.co.uk/uploads/Teenage_Pregnancy_Next_Steps_For_LAs_And_PCTs.pdf (accessed August 2012).

Department of Health (2009) *Healthy Child Programme: Pregnancy and the First Five Years of Life*. Available from: www.gov.uk/government/uploads/system/uploads/attachment_data/file/167998/Health_Child_Programme.pdf (accessed September 2013).

Department of Health (2011a) *No Health without Mental Health: A Cross Government Mental Health Outcomes Strategy for People of all Ages*. Available from: www.dh.gov.uk/en/Publicationsandstatistics/Publications/PublicationsPolicyAndGuidance/DH_123766 (accessed August 2012).

Department of Health (2011b) *Consultation on Preventing Suicide in England*. Available from: www.dh.gov.uk/prod_consum_dh/groups/dh_digitalassets/documents/digitalasset/dh_128463.pdf (accessed August 2012).

Department of Health and Department for Education (2004) *National Service Framework for Children, Young People and Maternity Services*. London: DH and DfE.

Dogra, N. and Leighton, S. (2009) *Nursing in Child and Adolescent Mental Health*. Maidenhead: Open University Press.

Dogra, N., Parkin, A., Gale, F. and Frake, C. (2009) *A Multidisciplinary Handbook of Child and Adolescent Mental Health for Front-line Professionals*, 2nd edn. London: Jessica Kingsley.

Fairburn, C.G. and Harrison, P. (2003) Eating Disorders. *The Lancet*, 361: 407–16.

Fazel, S. (2008) *Poor Mental Health Found among Young Offenders*. University of Oxford. Available from: www.ox.ac.uk/media/news_stories/2008/080903.html (accessed July 2013).

Gardner, F. (2001) *Self-harm: A Psychotherapeutic Approach*. Hove: Routledge.

Gaughan, M. (2011) Early Onset Psychosis. In Claveirole, A. and Gaughan, M. (eds) *Understanding Children and Young People's Mental Health*. Chichester: Wiley-Blackwell, pp.165–90.

Grundy, M. (2008) *The Worcester Journal*. Available from: www.worcesternews.co.uk/archive/2008/02/11/2033956.February_9_16/ (accessed July 2013).

Harrington, R. (2003) Depression and Suicidal Behaviour. In D. H. Skuse (ed.) *Child Psychology and Psychiatry An Introduction*. Oxford: The Medicine Publishing Co, pp. 125–28.

Hawton, K., Townsend, E., Appleby, L., Gunnell, D., Bennewith, O. and Cooper, J. (2001) Effects of Legislation Restricting Pack Sizes of Paracetamol and Salicylate on Self-poisoning in the UK: Before and after Study. *British Medical Journal*, 19 May 2001. Available from: www.bmj.com/content/322/7296/1203 (accessed July 2013).

Henry, B., Casp, A., Moffitt, T. and Silva, P. (1996) Temperamental and Familial Predictors of Violent and Non-violent Criminal Convictions from 3–18. *Developmental Psychopathology*, 32: 614–23. Available from: http://psycnet.apa.org/journals/dev/32/4/614/ (accessed November 2013).

Hider, P. (1998) *Youth Suicide Prevention by Primary Healthcare Professionals*. Christchurch, New Zealand: New Zealand Health Technology Assessment Clearing House. Available from: www.otago.ac.nz/christchurch/otago014022.pdf (accessed August 2012).

HM Government (2012) *Preventing Suicide in England: A Cross Government Outcome Strategy to Save Lives*. London: HM Government. Available from: www.gov.uk/government/uploads/system/uploads/attachment_data/file/216928/Preventing-Suicide-in-England-A-cross-government-outcomes-strategy-to-save-lives.pdf (accessed July 2013).

James, A.C. (2003) Bipolar Disorder. In D.H. Skuse (ed.) *Child Psychology and Psychiatry*. Oxford: The Medicine Publishing Co, pp. 121–4.

Jones, L. and Claveirole, A. (2011) ADHD. In Claveirole, A. and Gaughan, M. (eds) *Understanding Children and Young People's Mental Health*. Chichester: Wiley-Blackwell, pp. 191–216.

Karr-Morse, R. and Wiley, M. (1997) *Ghosts from the Nursery: Tracing the Roots of Violence*. New York: Atlantic Monthly Press.

Keenan, T. and Evans, S. (2009) *An Introduction to Child Development*. London: Sage.

Kendall, P.C. (2000) *Childhood Disorders*. Hove: Psychology Press.

Lask, B. (2003) *Practical Child Psychiatry: The Clinicians Guide*. London: BMJ Publishing Group.

Lask, B., Frampton, I. and Nunn, K. (2012) Anorexia Nervosa – A Noradrenergic Dysregulation Hypothesis. *Medical Hypotheses*, 78 (5): 580–4.

Lawrence, M. (2008) *The Anorexic Mind*. London: Karnac.

Lemma, A. (2010) *Under the Skin: A Psychoanalytic Study of Body Modification*. London: Routledge.

McDougall, J. (1989) *Theatres of the Body: A Psychoanalytical Approach to Psychosomatic Illness*. London: Free Association Books.

Main, M. and Solomon, J. (1986) Discovery of an Insecure-Disorganized/Disoriented Attachment Pattern. *Affective Development in Infancy*. Westport, CT: Ablex Publishing, pp. 95–124.

Mental Health Foundation (2006) *Truth Hurts Report of the National Inquiry into Self Harm Among Young People*. Available from: www.mentalhealth.org.uk/content/assets/PDF/publications/truth_hurts.pdf?view=Standard (accessed August 2012).

Mickel, A. (2009) Suicide Watch Bridgend Suicides the Lessons Learnt. *Community Care*. Available from: www.communitycare.co.uk/Articles/21/07/2009/112140/Bridgend-suicides-the-lessons-learnt.htm (accessed August 2012).

Mind (2012) *Understanding Borderline Personality Disorder*. Available from: www.mind.org.uk/assets/0002/1635/Understanding_bpd_2012.pdf (accessed September 2013).

Moffitt, T.E., Caspi, A., Harrington, H. and Milne, B.J. (2002) Males on the Life Course Persistent and Adolescence-limited Antisocial Pathways: Follow up at Age 26. *Developmental Psychopathology*, 14 (1): 179–207. Available from: journals.cambridge.org/action/displayFulltext?type=1&fid=100938&jid=DPP&volumeId=14&issueId=01&aid=100937 (accessed August 2013).

Muggleton, J. (2012) *Raising Martians – From Crash Landing to Leaving Home: How to Help a Child with Asperger Syndrome or High-functioning Autism*. London: Jessica Kingsley.

National Autistic Society (2013) *What is Autism?* Available from: www.autism.org.uk/about-autism/autism-and-asperger-syndrome-an-introduction/what-is-autism.aspx (accessed August 2013).

National Collaborating Centre for Mental Health (2009) *ADHD: The NICE Guideline on Diagnosis and Management of ADHD in Children, Young People and Adults*. London: The British Psychological Society and the Royal College of Psychiatrists.

National Institute for Clinical Excellence (2002) *Scope*. Available from: www.nice.org.uk/nicemedia/pdf/Self-HarmScopeFinalV3140502.pdf (accessed July 2013).

National Institute for Clinical Excellence (2006) *Bipolar Disorder: The Management of Bipolar Disorder in Adults, Children and Adolescents in Primary and Secondary Care*. Available from: www.nice.org.uk/nicemedia/pdf/CG38niceguideline.pdf (accessed August 2012).

National Institute for Clinical Excellence (2008) *Attention Deficit Hyperactivity Disorder: Diagnosis and Management of ADHD in Children, Young People and Adults*. Available from: www.nice.org.uk/nicemedia/live/12061/42059/42059.pdf (accessed August 2013).

National Institute for Clinical Excellence (2009) *Borderline Personality Disorder: Treatment and Management*. Available from: www.nice.org.uk/nicemedia/live/12125/42900/42900. pdf (accessed September 2013).

National Institute for Clinical Excellence (2011) *Psychosis with Coexisting Substance Misuse: Assessment and Management in Adults and Young People*. Available from: www.nice.org. uk/nicemedia/live/13414/53729/53729.pdf (accessed August 2013).

National Institute for Clinical Excellence (2013) *Antisocial Behaviour and Conduct Disorders in Children and Young People: Recognition, Intervention and Management*. Available from: www.nice.org.uk/nicemedia/live/14116/63310/63310.pdf (accessed August 2013).

National Scientific Council on the Developing Child (2004) *Children's Emotional Development is Built into the Architecture of Their Brains*, Working Paper No. 2, Center on the Developing Child, Harvard University, USA. Available from: www.developingchild. net (accessed July 2013).

NSPCC (2009) *Young People who Self-harm: Implications for Public Health Practitioners*. Available from: www.nspcc.org.uk/Inform/research/briefings/youngpeoplewhoselfharm-pdf_wdf63294.pdf (accessed August 2012).

Nunn, K. (2013) The Sensitivities that Hinder and the Sensitivities that Heal. In Lask, B. and Bryant-Waugh, R. (eds) *Eating Disorders in Childhood and Adolescence*, 4th edn. London: Routledge, pp. 3–11.

O'Connor, R., Rasmussen, S., Miles, J. and Hawton, K. (2009) Self-harm in Adolescents: Self Report Survey in Schools in Scotland. *British Journal of Psychiatry*, 194: 68–72. Available from: bjp.rcpsych.org/content/194/1/68.full (accessed July 2013).

Pearce, J. (2004) Emotional Disorders in Young People. In Aggleton, P., Hurry, J. and Warwick, I. (eds) *Young People and Mental Health*. Chichester: Wiley-Blackwell, pp. 47–72.

Piccinelli, M. and Wilkinson, G. (2000) Gender Differences in Depression. *British Journal of Psychiatry*, (177): 486–92. Available from: http://bjp.rcpsych.org/content/177/6/486. full?sid=14c09e5a-1b4a-4931-aa79-db987459ea0d (accessed November 2013).

Preventing Suicide in England: A Cross Government Outcome Strategy to Save Lives (2012) Available from: www.gov.uk/government/uploads/system/uploads/attachment_data/file/216928/Preventing-Suicide-in-England-A-cross-government-outcomes-strategy-to-save-lives.pdf (accessed July 2013).

PSHE (2011) *Personal, Social and Health Education*. Available from: www.education.gov.uk/schools/teachingandlearning/curriculum/primary/b00199209/pshe (accessed August 2012).

Royal College of Psychiatrists (2002) *Department of Health Suicide Prevention Strategy for England: College Response*. London: Royal College of Psychiatrists.

Royal College of Psychiatrists (2012a) *Mental Health and Growing Up, Fourth Edition; Self-harm in Young People: Information for Parents, Carers and Anyone who Works with Young People*. Available from: www.rcpsych.ac.uk/mentalhealthinformation/mentalhealthand-growingup (accessed August 2012).

Royal College of Psychiatrists (2012b) *Cannabis and Mental Health*. Available from: www.rcpsych.ac.uk/mentalhealthinfo/youngpeople/cannabis.aspx (accessed August 2012).

Royal College of Psychiatrists (2012c) *Mental Health and Growing Up, Fourth Edition; Alcohol and Drugs: What Parents Need to Know*. Available from: www.rcpsych.ac.uk/mentalhealth-info/mentalhealthandgrowingup/alcoholdrugsparents.aspx (accessed August 2012).

Rutter, M. (1985) Resilience in the Face of Adversity: Protective Factors and Resistance to Psychiatric Disorders. *British Journal of Psychiatry*, 147: 589–611.

Rutter, M. (2006) Implications of Resilience Concepts for Scientific Understanding. *Annals of the New York Academy of Science*, 1094: 1–12.

Schofield, G., Ward, E., Biggart, L., Scaife, V., Dodsworth, J., Larsson, B., Haynes, A. and Stone, N. (2012) *Looked After Children and Offending*. Centre for Research on the Child and Family, University of East Anglia. Available from: www.tactcare.org.uk/data/files/resources/52/lac_and_offending_reducing_risk_promoting_resilience_fullreport_200212.pdf (accessed August 2012).

SEAL (2010) *Social and Emotional Aspects of Learning*. Available from: www.education.gov.uk/publications/standard/publicationDetail/Page1/DFE-RR049 (accessed August 2012).

Silver, L.B. (1990) Attention Deficit-Hyperactivity Disorder: Is it a Learning Disability or a Related Disorder? *Journal of Learning Disabilities*, 23 (7): 394–7.

Stice, E. (2002) Risk and Maintenance Factors for Eating Pathology: A Meta-analytic Review. *Psychological Bulletin,* 128(5): 825–48.

Street, C., Anderson, Y. and Plumb, J. (2007) *Maintaining the Momentum: Towards Excellent Services for Children and Young People's Mental Health*. London: NHS Confederation.

Strober, M., Schmidt-Lackner, S., Freeman, R., Bower, S., Lampert, C. and DeAntionio, M. (1999) Recovery and Relapse in Adolescents with Bipolar Affective Illness: A Five Year Naturalistic, Prospective Follow-up. *Journal American Academy Child Adolescent Psychiatry*, 34(6): 724–31.

Together We Stand: The Commissioning, Role and Management of CAMHS, Health Advisory Service Report. (1995) London: HMSO.

Treasure, J. and Alexander, J. (2013) *Anorexia Nervosa: A Recovery Guide for Sufferers, Families and Friends*. London: Routledge.

Treasure, J. and Karwautz, A. (2004) Eating Disorders. In Aggleton, P. Hurry, J. and Warwick, I. (eds) *Young People and Mental Health*. Chichester: Wiley-Blackwell, pp. 73.

Vostanis, P. (2007) Mental Health and Mental Disorders. In Coleman, F. and Hagell, A. (eds) *Adolescence Risk and Resilience: Against the Odds*. Chichester: John Wiley, pp. 89–107.

Waddell, M. (2002) *Inside Lives: Psychoanalysis and the Growth of the Personality*. London: Karnac.

Wing, L. (1996) *The Autistic Spectrum*. London: Constable.

World Health Organization (2012) *Risks to Mental Health An Overview of Vulnerabilities and Risk Factors*, Geneva, Switzerland, World Health Organization, available from: www.who.int/mental_health/mhgap/risks_to_mental_health_EN_27_08_12.pdf (accessed November 2013).

World Health Organization (2013) *International Classification of Diseases 10 (ICD 10)*. Available from: www.who.int/classifications/icd/en/ (accessed July 2013).

Zubin, J. and Spring, B. (1977) Vulnerability: A New View of Schizophrenia. *Journal of Abnormal Psychology*, 86 (2): 103–26.

2

INFANT, CHILD AND ADOLESCENT DEVELOPMENT

MADDIE BURTON

Overview

- What does 'development' mean?
- The nature versus nurture debate
- What is child development theory and who were the theorists?
- Developmental theories discussed
- Family and parenting influences on development
- Application of theory

INTRODUCTION

This chapter is a brief introduction to child development. The aim is to convey a flavour of the many theories which act as a mirror to the complexity of understanding and knowledge surrounding child development. There is no single approach to be taken; rather we are bringing together a set of ideas. What feels most relevant today to the context of child and adolescent mental health is to sample an eclectic mix from a combination of psychoanalytic, attachment and ecological systems theories. Key aspects of these theories are that healthy optimal development is dependent on the quality and consistency of relationships both within and outside the family.

Gerhardt (2004) calls it: *building a brain*. No other organ takes so long to mature. In the last decade theoretical models have moved from cognition as a central theme in development to a psychobiological model being at the fore. Schore (2005) suggests that the attainment of an attachment bond of emotional communication represents key events in infancy, more so than the development of complex cognitions. This is due to the self-regulatory mechanisms which are located in the right hemisphere of the developing brain. Evidence from neuroscience now shows that the architecture of the brain is built on this foundation and confirms the significance of the role of attachment theories (National Scientific Council on the Developing Child, 2004b).

At the heart we are considering and thinking of human *beings*; all of us born into a world and a complexity of relationships and most significantly a first relationship which starts to inform us as a *being*. Becoming a *person* involves a large investment by others early in life and an emerging sense of self as reflected back to us through the eyes and minds of others. Music (2011: 7) tells us that:

> ... a person's sense of self arises from being in the minds of others, without which it simply does not develop ... and that one's sense of self is socially and co-constructed.

WHAT DOES 'DEVELOPMENT' MEAN?

Development can be viewed as 'patterns of change' beginning at conception and continuing throughout life. It can be seen as a path or journey with different milestones or transitions that need to be travelled and accomplished. At each milestone or transition point, certain developmental tasks have to be negotiated and worked through in order to proceed to the next point or stage. You will often hear professional and clinical terminology in use such as: 'has met (or not met) developmental milestones'. If points can be managed successfully, the next transition point will be easier to negotiate and pass through. Sometimes hurdles and obstructions can and will appear on the way, leading to a requirement for renegotiation. At times individuals can get stuck at a particular stage. Similarly throughout life, changes in circumstances and emotional upheaval can precipitate an individual to revert to earlier stages which perhaps had not been worked through during their child development processes. There can be ongoing movement in and out of these developmental phases or 'states of mind'. An older adult may have the state of mind of a child or a child the state of mind of an older person for moments or periods of time. Waddell (2002) aptly describes the present, past and future as being contained in any one state of mind using some interesting examples in her book.

Negotiating developmental tasks can be seen when we think about parallels between 'toddler' and 'adolescent' behaviour. The phrase 'toddler tantrums', as a description of difficult behaviour is commonly cited. Similarly adolescent behaviour is sometimes seen as unpopular or difficult to accept or 'socially unacceptable'. Both of these age groups have to negotiate an emerging sense of self and 'states of mind'. There are some similar transition themes of individuation and identity formation. The toddler is negotiating becoming more independent and no longer a 'baby'.

The adolescent has to negotiate leaving childhood and becoming an adult. These are huge developmental tasks and transitions to undertake; why would they and how could they be expected to run smoothly? Yet there are often higher expectations of 'behaviour' at these times for both age groups.

There are however differences in cultures and expectations around development. For example adolescence is now considered a relatively long process in the western developed world, although in previous centuries this has not always been the case. In Britain today, as part of the developed world, there are subtle changes emerging with more young people remaining longer at home and in compulsory education; changes driven by economic factors, coexisting with social and political change. In the developing world there is a different economic imperative such as a need to contribute to the family economy. In that world young people move quickly into adulthood with a relatively short adolescent phase and a much shorter time spent in education. This would have also been the case in Britain prior to the 20th century. It is also worth considering that 'normal' child development theories originate in a western context without perhaps appropriate consideration for variations in cultures. Theories have tended to develop as a reflection and response to events and the historic period of time and social context where they were considered. It is widely understood that *attachment theory* is a universal concept regardless of context and culture. Children with disabilities may not meet 'normal development' milestones. It can be unhelpful to define their developmental progress according to 'normal' milestones (Lindon, 2010).

Human development can be considered as taking place within the domains of:

- Biological or physical changes such as birth, growth and puberty.
- Emotional (understanding and experience): learning to recognise and manage feelings.
- Social (relationships): forming and maintaining relationships, managing transitions.
- Cognitive (thought processes): developing language, learning to read, problem solving.

Whilst the separate domains are recognised, they all are interdependent and influential on and of each other with neither existing in isolation. Physical and psychological growth is a long drawn out process for humans providing added time and opportunity to acquire complex skills and knowledge necessary for inhabiting and managing a complex social world. It is not just about a set of maturational processes operating independently from environmental influences.

NATURE VERSUS NURTURE

Nature or nurture has been one of the most controversial and debated areas in child development theory. What is the underlying driver of development? Is it *nature*, an inborn pattern, or is it *nurture*, driven by the impact of experience and environment? It is largely agreed today that neither position operates in a sole capacity but rather it is about what the child brings in terms of temperament and genetic characteristics (*nature*) and how these articulate with the environment and experiences (*nurture*). The combination of *nature and nurture* co-creates the child, the human being, the person. According to the *nature* theory developmental changes are predetermined and controlled by a set of genetic instructions which are universal to all children with no cultural boundaries and are impervious to environmental influences (Gesell, 1925, cited in Bee and Boyd, 2010). Spelke (1991) suggested that babies are born with pre-existing conceptions of response patterns and that such bias limits and constrains the amount of developmental pathways. Behaviour geneticists have endeavoured to show that cognitive abilities, children's temperaments and aspects of pathological behaviour are genetically influenced. Development is considered to be sequential; a pattern of emerging characteristics or skills, and that parents have little influence on child development (Harris, 2009, cited in Music, 2011: 2).

The *nurture* theory suggests experience plays a large part and that the timing of experiences and the interaction with maturational or developmental patterns are complex and crucial. Postwar views held that individuals were blank slates and could be moulded by parental and other external influences (Pinker, 2002, cited in Music, 2011: 2).

Further, gene/environment interaction considers that a child inherits his/her genes from the parents who create the child's environment, so influence is two-fold. In addition inherited qualities and temperament affect the way the child is responded to and his/her subsequent reactions (Reiss, 1998). Studies have led theorists to suggest that each child inherits characteristics which make them both vulnerable (risk factors) and resilient (protective factors). For example a child may be genetically predisposed (*nature*) to developing attention deficit hyperactivity disorder (ADHD). There may be other family members with a diagnosis. With the combination of a poor environment in terms of either abuse or attachment difficulties (*nurture*), the child may then develop ADHD (Music, 2011). Similarly a young person may be genetically predisposed to clinical depression or psychosis, which does not in itself mean the condition will necessarily develop. However, if there is a combination of other negative external factors, depression, psychosis or other significant mental illness may emerge and develop into a clinical condition. The result, in both cases, is a combination and interaction between genetic inheritance or predisposition (*nature*) and environmental experiences which act as triggers (*nurture*) in influencing development. It is now generally accepted that both nature and nurture play an important role in development (Rutter, 2002). Children are born with a unique genetic inheritance and temperament; the key to development is the interplay with *how the environment is experienced* which creates the inner reality, the person (Diem-Wille, 2011). In a family siblings may share similar experiences yet each individual sibling will respond in a different way to varying degrees, albeit it within similar patterns. Music's (2011) *Nurturing Natures* tells us that:

> ... human life develops from the delicate interplay of nature and nurture, the meeting of a bundle of inherited potentials and the cultural, social and personal influences of the adults in an infant's life. (Music, 2011: 24)

Early environmental experiences are critical to the maturation of the brain. Nature's potential can only be realised if it is facilitated by nurture (Schore, 2005: 205).

CHILD DEVELOPMENT THEORY AND THEORISTS

All theories comprise a set of ideas on how children develop according to and *in relation* to various internal and external influences and experiences. There are many common threads in the various theories, although individually they are each quite distinct. Each has a different emphasis and places importance on different aspects of growth. Child development theories both past and present have a direct influence on social policy and practice in areas of education, health and child rearing.

Briefly, and later in more detail, child development theories included in the chapter come from the following fields.

Psychodynamic theories

'*Psyche*' literally meaning: mind, emotion, spirit, self. '*Dynamic*': being an attempt to explain *how* the personality works and develops. The idea is that unconscious and conscious thoughts influence behaviour. Development is seen as stages or tasks which have to be negotiated and are experienced as *conflict*. Early life experiences are viewed as central to the development of the personality.

Main theorists: initially Sigmund Freud. Then followed by his daughter Anna Freud, and Melanie Klein and Erik Erikson. These theorists made initial connections with each other and they laid the foundations of thinking about child development and children as a separate entity for the first time rather than just being included with adults. The foundation they laid has continually been added to and their early work was followed by other theorists including Wilfred Bion (container/contained) and Donald Winnicott (object relations theory). Psychodynamic theories continued to develop despite two of the original theorists, Klein and Anna Freud, disagreeing over their theories and agreeing to dissociate with each other. Today child psychoanalysts will consider themselves to be either 'Kleinian' or 'Freudian' or even 'Winnicottian', as Donald Winnicott and others sought to hold a middle ground and develop relational or object relations theory which connected social constructivism and psychoanalytical theories. Colwyn Trevarthen (intersubjectivity) and Daniel Stern (infant development) also made important contributions in the latter part of the 20th century. Peter Fonagy (mentalisation) and others have continued today to develop and support psychodynamic theories as a way of understanding and making sense of child development and the important links to emotional health and wellbeing.

Attachment theories

These propose that children use adults as a safe haven and secure base which is also safe and comfortable and from which the world can be explored. *Attachment quality* is seen as crucial for healthy development as are food and nutrition, and that emotional care is equally essential. Attachment *type* or *quality* is a predictor of all future relationship patterns across the life span.

Main theorists: John Bowlby and Mary Ainsworth.

Behavioural learning theories

These originated from studies with animals. The focus is on children learning through experience and that childhood behaviours are subject to change and modification according to patterns of reward and punishment. Terminology includes *classical, operant conditioning* and *reinforcement*. Behaviourists considered behaviour could be modified according to conditioning experiences as the human baby was considered a 'blank slate'.

Main theorists: Ivan Pavlov, John Watson and Burrhus Skinner.

Social learning theories

These are also behaviourist theories and include terminology such as: *conditioning, observation and reinforcement*. Children develop by observing adults and other children, modelling behaviours. Social learning theories also began to be known as social cognitive theories (Lindon, 2010).

Main theorist: Albert Bandura.

Ecological systems theory

Ecology can also be thought about as *context* and since the late 1970s and 1980s there has been a drive to move beyond thinking about the immediate family and environment (where the focus had previously been on the maternal relationship) and to consider the impact of the wider context on development. Children grow up in complex social environments which are embedded in larger social and political systems.

Main theorist: Urie Bronfenbrenner.

Cognitive theories

Cognitive theories place the greatest importance on cognitive rather than personality development. The focus is on how a child makes sense of his/her experience and interaction with the environment. Piaget believed that children are active participants in their cognitive development, but unlike Piaget, Vygotsky viewed social interaction and context as being intrinsic factors. Cultural influences added further dimensions which the child would not be able to achieve in isolation. Vygotsky attempted to create a theory, taking into account the interaction between all factors with the belief we can only be understood within our social and historical contexts. There are similarities between Vygotsky's theory and Bronfenbrenner's ecological systems theory. Piaget and Vygotsky have influenced education practice both in the past and currently.

Main theorists: Jean Piaget and Lev Vygotsky.

PSYCHODYNAMIC THEORIES

Sigmund Freud (1856–1939)

Freud is considered the 'father' of psychoanalysis and psychodynamic theory originates with him and has continued to evolve and develop variants located with other theorists. The original principles remain. His theory of human personality posited that development occurs from a balance between unconscious drives and the conscious need to adapt to the environment. Development occurs in stages viewed as tasks or conflicts. Freud believed that early experience is central to the development of the personality. He identified and proposed that personality is comprised of three structures:

- *Id:* instinctive drives operating according to the pleasure principle; Freud proposed the id dominates a child's behaviour.
- *Ego:* conscious part of personality, satisfies drives in a more socially acceptable manner, about perception, logical thinking, problem solving and memory.
- *Superego:* results from an incorporation of parental and societal values, the conscience, can be negative and punishing, also positive and rewarding.

He suggested the ego becomes the arbitrator between the id and the superego.

Freud proposed the existence of an unconscious sexual drive or libido and that through *defence mechanisms* unconscious material is created over time. He proposed *defence mechanisms* develop when the anxiety created by threats from the internal and external worlds cannot be resolved by any rational thinking processes. Defence mechanisms therefore reduce anxiety and include:

Denial: acting as though a problem does not exist, so turning a blind eye.

Repression: forgetting something painful ... into the subconscious.

Projection: attributing something to another whilst not acknowledging it for ourselves.

Introjection: reverse of projection (can be a positive and essential part of development).

Regression: reverting to an earlier developmental stage, e.g. perhaps having a tantrum when you are not a toddler or thumb sucking for comfort (oral stage), when faced with a new situation which provokes anxiety.

Displacement: expressing feelings to another object rather than the one provoking the initial reaction, e.g. kicking the door or the dog.

Rationalisation: explaining a way out rather than accepting the true situation.

Reaction formation: experiencing/expressing the opposite feelings to what is really felt.

Idealisation: avoiding the acknowledgement of negative feelings and elevating the positive status.

Intellectualisation: focusing on intellectual rather than emotional responses.

Splitting: a combination of projection and denial, e.g. hating the person you love.

Fixation: inability to develop emotionally beyond a certain point, either through fear of the next stage or because the current stage has not been achieved.

Activity

Can you identify any defence mechanisms? These will be about maintaining self-image and protecting the mind from anxiety. Consider aspects of your personality you feel strongly about and what you may be defending yourself from.

Freud also identified *psychosexual stages* which were focused on maturation with each stage revolving around sexual impulses or libido, seen as an essential part of personality development:

- *Oral stage, 0–1 year:* baby experiences pleasure/displeasure focusing on behaviours around the mouth, e.g. sucking, biting and chewing.
- *Anal stage, 1–3 years:* pleasure focused on elimination, conflict may emerge as a result of parents' attempt to toilet train.
- *Phallic stage, 3–5 years:* pleasure/difficulties focused on genital area, children have to manage sexual attraction towards the parent of the opposite sex which is resolved by identification with the same sex parent. These conflicts Freud referred to as the Oedipus complex. Freud suggested that boys fear castration by their fathers due to sexual feelings towards their mothers, while girls experience penis envy.
- *Latency stage, 5–onset of puberty:* sexual drives are repressed and the focus is on developing intellectual and social skills.
- *Genital stage and adolescence,* begins in puberty and continues throughout life: sexual impulses previously repressed during latency re-emerge in response to the biological upheaval of puberty. Sexual impulses become intensified during this stage and are now directed towards peers (Bee and Boyd, 2010: 245).

It is important to remember that while Freud's theories may sound a little unusual to us today, they were first introduced in a time period dominated by the behaviourists such as Pavlov, Watson and Skinner.

Erik Erikson (1902–94)

Erikson emphasised the role of identity, social and cultural factors as opposed to Freud's sexual and aggressive drives (Bee and Boyd, 2010: 246). He proposed a life span developmental theory with eight stages (Table 2.1). His theory is sometimes referred to as the eight stages of man. At each stage a crisis (age-related task) has to be negotiated; how successfully this is resolved or not will impact on further development. Crucially, Erikson felt that successful development involves achieving the right balance in and at each stage.

Table 2.1 Erikson's 'eight stages of man'

Trust vs mistrust	Birth–1 year	Developing trust in carers, self and the environment
Autonomy vs shame and doubt	1–3 years	Developing a sense of independence
Initiative vs guilt	3–6 years	Control over environment, identification with parents
Industry vs inferiority	6 years–adolescence	'I am what I learn'; developing social and intellectual skills
Identity vs identity diffusion	Adolescence: up to 20 years	Understanding who you are, by integrating what has been learnt so far and identifying with like-minded groups
Intimacy vs isolation	Young adulthood: 20–40 years	Developing intimate and stable relationships
Generativity vs stagnation	Middle adulthood: 40–60 years	Developing ways to avoid feelings of stagnation; continuing psychological growth
Integrity vs despair	60 years +	Evaluating your life and integration

Wilfred Bion (1897–1979)

Bion further extended the work of Melanie Klein. Bion concentrated on the relationship and the mind's capacity for emotional development. His work became known as 'post-Kleinian thinking'.

Bion considered the quality of the original communication between mother and baby was very important. Mother brings a 'thinking' self; a capacity for *reverie*. The mother becomes the *container* and a model for processing emotional experience. So initially the mother 'thinks' for the infant, thereafter the infant will be able to think for him/herself, and later mother will think with the infant. Bion felt emotional experience was at the core of development. He also pioneered working in groups with adults and group 'states of mind' (Mawson, 2012). Bion's theories influence models of practice today. The Solihull Approach parenting strategy includes Bion's concept of containment (Douglas, 2007).

Anna Freud (1895–1982)

Anna was one of Sigmund Freud's daughters and worked with him closely. Anna set up the 'war nurseries' in London in 1941. She was interested in observing the children and working with them and also involving parents, which was unusual for the time. Children were based in 'family groups' with the nursery staff where they could receive a consistent continuity of care and be able to form consistent attachments with each other. Anna promoted understanding of the child's perspective and child development and with Melanie Klein was one of the founders of child psychoanalysis. The Hampstead Clinic she founded in 1952 was dedicated to therapy for children and families, training in child therapy as distinct from adult training, the application of psychoanalytic theory to education, social and legal reform and research based on detailed observation. Many of Anna's original ideas from her observations and understanding of the impact of stress and separation from parents have influenced the caring of children today. The clinic was renamed the Anna Freud Centre following her death in 1982 and continues the work Anna started, dedicated to children's emotional wellbeing (Anna Freud Centre, 2013).

Donald Winnicott (1896–1971)

Donald Winnicott was a consultant paediatrician who following years of his own analysis qualified as a psychoanalyst in 1934. He would later become the first man to qualify as a child analyst. He combined his long 40-year paediatric career with the psychoanalytic treatment of adults and children in a London hospital. Winnicott focused more on emotional life and the meaning and formative effects of early relationships, which he called *object relations*: this stresses the primary significance of the nature and quality of the relationship between the self and another. Winnicott felt that parental environmental factors were what contributed to the infant's developing internal world. Winnicott stated:

> ... there's no such thing as an infant ... if you show me the baby you certainly show me someone caring for the baby. (Winnicott, 1956: 303)

Winnicott defined this phase as one of '*absolute dependence*'. If there were early environment failures, long-term results could be catastrophic and that psychopathology is a consequence of early parental failure. Object relations develop in a context of a relationship that starts with parents and the internalised representations as a result of this relationship, which then continues to influence relationships throughout life as mental representations of the self and others (object). Winnicott (1956) also coined the phrase '*good enough mothering*', meaning if parenting is just that, an optimal developmental outcome could be realised. No one gets it right all of the time.

ATTACHMENT THEORY

John Bowlby (1907–90) combined ethology (the study of behaviour) and psychodynamic theory, creating *attachment* theory. He was caught between Freud and Klein in an attempt to increase the scientific status of child development theory and to consider the role of the environment in developmental theory. Bowlby hoped to reconcile differences but with no success. However his work on attachment theory, with Mary Ainsworth, has now achieved the scientific status he originally set out to secure. Emerging research from the neuroscience field concurs with Bowlby's original assertions and acknowledges the importance of *affect regulation*, which can only achieve optimum significance within a secure attachment relationship. If the brain is developing within a relationship of a care giver that is providing sensitive, responsible care giving, the brain can be modulated early on in terms of regulation.

Bowlby identified attachment theory as a fundamental behaviour that was distinct from feeding but no less important for survival. The attachment figure's equivalent tie to the child was termed the 'care giving bond'. Bowlby's original idea of attachment focused on the process of bonding and the impact of this process on psychological development. Studies beginning in the 1990s started to suggest that early bonding was not an all or nothing process, but that attachment continues to develop and strengthen throughout the early months of life and beyond (Goldberg et al., 2000).

It is important to remember the context of Bowlby and Ainsworth's early work. Along with Winnicott their research was primarily focused on the impact of separating children from a maternal figure. At the time many children were being evacuated from London and other cities during the blitz of the Second World War, either to homes in the safer countryside or into residential care. Bowlby compared the effects of institutionalised living versus family life; his assertions continue to this day. For example, the Children Act 1989 integrated the belief that 'bad homes are better than good institutions'. Today great efforts are made to ensure children can remain and continue to have connections with their birth family, despite child protection activity and children entering the looked after system. Bowlby's research and ideas around 'bonding' also influenced paediatric and obstetric practices, which resulted in changes in children's hospital settings, maternity hospitals and practice, in terms of keeping children, babies and mothers together.

Bowlby proposed that infants and small children have an innate need to seek proximity to their care givers and that this was an evolutionary mechanism for both animals and humans. He quotes William James: 'the great source of terror in infancy is solitude' (Howe, 2011: 6). For infants safety is about staying close. Therefore the attachment figure becomes the location when under threat and feeling fearful. Children who elicit care, by provoking the necessary responses in their care givers, will stand a greater chance of survival. This is about safety being internalised. An infant's principal care giver will become the attachment figure. The long-term effects of neglect, abandonment and prolonged separation should not be underestimated (Howe, 2011):

> All of us from the cradle to the grave, are happiest when life is organised as a series of excursions, long or short, from the secure base provided by our attachment figures. (Bowlby, 1988: 69)

Bowlby concluded from his studies that:

> ... the prolonged deprivation of a young child, of maternal care, may have grave and far reaching effects on his character and so on the whole of his future life. (Bowlby, 1952: 46)

Throughout life attachment can be seen as a primary mechanism for the regulation of relationships between humans (Schore, 2005).

Children develop other attachment figures with members of the extended family such as grandparents. These would be figures seen as reliable sources of safety and comfort. These may also include key workers in child care settings. The key worker model is now widespread practice in health, education and social care settings. So something is clear about the importance of 'relationship' and the emotional activity involved as a supportive factor. In England there is a requirement in the Early Years Foundation Stage to operate a key worker system (Lindon, 2010).

Using the example of my own granddaughter, who started preschool at age 2, initially she would find separation from mum, one of her primary attachment figures, upsetting. However she was helped to feel safe and secure at preschool by her key worker who would comfort her. According to my granddaughter, 'Pat' (the key worker) would share her toast and grapes with her or sit her on her lap for a special story. She soon settled at preschool and talks fondly of her key worker and the other staff. Her key worker (secondary attachment figure) would help her in feeling safe and secure when away from her primary attachment figures.

Other attachment figures or secondary attachment figures play an important protective role. Especially if there are temporary setbacks with a primary attachment figure, separation or hospitalisation for instance. One can imagine how potentially difficult it can be for children when primary care givers disappear for long periods or are absent through work commitments or a variety of reasons such as divorce and separation of the parents.

It is worth remembering that many of the theories already discussed have a preoccupation with the mother and infant dyad. Biologically mothers give birth to babies but there is also a father in the family system, therefore a triadic system and a paren-tal couple. What is crucial to the developing infant is the quality of the parental cou-ple relationship (Barrows, 2004). Attachment hierarchies exist with mothers *usually* being considered to be the primary attachment figure. Bowlby and other theorists modified their earlier conclusions with regard to the implications of maternal depri-vation. For example, when a child is looked after for part of the day by a known and trusted person other than a mother, then this does no harm: children will develop a hierarchy of attachment figures.

The attachment system becomes activated when under distress or threat, which in turn initiates attachment behaviours. The attachment figure's response to the infant is crucial and thus how the infant is helped or not helped to feel safe. If attachment behaviours, such as crying, do not achieve a response the attachment system remains activated as a survival mechanism and so there is less time for other developmental opportunities such as play and social inter-action. So for children exposed to ongoing neglect, abuse and rejection there is less time for play and developing relationships. If the parent's care giving system can be activated by the child then the child's attachment system can be deactivated. The time period for attachment quality to be realised is from the age of 6 months to 5 years, coinciding with a time of the most vulnerability and dependence (Howe, 2011: 18).

Mary Ainsworth classified attachment based on her research and what is known as 'The Strange Situation' experiment. It was about observation of the child's reac-tions during separations and subsequent reunions with the mother (or primary care giver). From this the type of *attachment quality* could be formulated: initially three attachment qualities were identified, two more were added later.

Secure attachment (Type B)

The child has a clear preference towards the mother (or primary care giver) over others. The care giver sensitively responds to the child's communications and the child is happy in their presence. There is distress shown by the child on separation but on reunion after reassurance the child settles again. *Secure attachment* predicts a better quality of parent–child relationship and other improved skills and positive emotions.

Anxious-avoidant (Type A)

Also known as '*insecure-avoidant*', the child appears aloof and shows minimal distress on separation, and on reuniting the care giver is ignored or avoided. The child does not seek contact and can be watchful and wary. Play is minimised and there is little discrimination between care givers and strangers. The child has learnt to minimise his or her attachment needs and has developed a pattern of avoiding an attachment behaviour to avoid rejection.

Anxious-ambivalent (Type C)

Also referred to as *'insecure-ambivalent'* or *'resistant'*, here attachment appears strong but is not secure. The child is distressed on separation but does not settle on reunion. So despite the care giver returning, separation anxiety continues. Anxious-ambivalent children are often the result of inconsistent parenting styles which sometimes are hostile and rejecting with a lack of empathy for the child.

All of the above categories of secure, anxious-avoidant and anxious-ambivalent are classified as organised, meaning that there is a behavioural adaption within the care giving environment. Each pattern adopted organises attachment behaviour to achieve the goal of maintaining and increasing attachment to the primary care giver in times of need and danger (Howe, 2011: 45).

Disorganised attachment (Type D)

Disorganised attachment happens when the carer is viewed as frightening and unavailable as a source of comfort or reassurance. In abusive situations the carer can be both a source of danger and comfort. Children may display the need to be held but will look away and avoid eye contact. Children may show a confused mix of ambivalent and avoidant responses including strange behaviours such as repetitive movements (e.g. rocking) and frozen responses on separation and confused responses to the care giver on reunion. These children experience relationships with care givers as stressful. Consequently their attachment systems remain in a chronic state of activation with unregulated arousal states (Howe, 2011: 47).

Even very young babies will look away and avoid eye contact from an intrusive or frightening face. Disorganised attachment leaves the child with nothing to draw on; the external experiences have an enduring significance throughout life and are most likely to produce long-term behavioural and mental health problems. This is most prevalent in families where there are serious difficulties combined with low socioeconomic status.

Non-attached

This category relates to children who have not formed any attachments. A prime example would be children in institutional care where there is a lack of opportunity for building personal relationships even with staff. This has been seen in recent times in the children from the Romanian orphanages. These children have serious problems in social relationships and have impaired cognitive development (Beckett and Taylor, 2010: 53).

Attachment has a biological origin and function in terms of brain development and survival (*nature*). The quality of attachment is determined by experiences in the environment (*nurture*), which predicts future relationship patterns as a lifelong process.

Internal working models

Once attachment is established an *internal working model* or *mental representation* is created through an individual's experience during infancy, and the impact and inter-relation of the responses to and from others and the self, usually by age 5 (Bee and Boyd, 2010). It is not necessarily defined by life events but rather, about the quality of the way one is looked after in infancy which then builds a *capacity* for what life may throw at the individual. The link with attachment is that different attachment qualities or styles in conjunction with the internal working model produce different emotional responses according to individual variations. Internal models of experience look at the importance of the individual's perception of their experience, which is based on a core set of beliefs about the world, the individual and others. These are originally based on early experiences but once they are developed into an internal model they go on to form the basis of how future life events and relationships are perceived (Epstein, 1991, cited in Bee and Boyd, 2010). In turn events and perception of relationships reinforce the internal working model.

There is some equivalence between internal working models (Bowlby) and object relations theory (Winnicott) in that both assume perceptions of the self in relation to others in terms of relationships. These are some of the most important aspects of human development (Calabrese et al., 2005).

With Bowlby, Anna Freud and Winnicott were instrumental in influencing changes around the care of infants and children and of keeping families together and under-standing the disabling aspects of trauma when children are separated from care givers. Many of their observations and work took place during the evacuations of children under stress, to avoid the bombings during the Second World War. Their legacy is seen today in hospital and healthcare settings where parents can now remain with their sick children. In education the whole Early Years provision is about preparing and introducing children to school, and reducing the potential trauma of sudden separation. Their work is as relevant today as when it was first published (Winnicott, 2012).

BEHAVIOURAL LEARNING THEORIES

The main behavioural learning theorists were Pavlov, Watson and Skinner, who worked on developing their theories at the end of the 19th century and early part of the 20th century. Aspects of their theories continue today, particularly in institutional, educational and Early Years settings.

Ivan Pavlov (1849–1936) was a Russian biologist working with dogs. He presented food at the same time as a sound so over time the dogs gradually associated the sound with food and eventually salivated when they heard the sound. His theory became known as *classical conditioning*. Similarly, pairing of unrelated words with words with an unpleasant meaning creates an unpleasant reaction to the original word. This model shows how everyday sounds and smells can be turned into traumatic stimuli because they were associated with the traumatic event (Gibson, 2006). Classical conditioning lies behind many phobias and is about learning associations.

They are always about an experience of an event, something which has happened. So a fear of flying in an aircraft is not as a result of classical conditioning (unless the person had survived a plane crash).

Activity

Develop a case scenario explaining the link between classical conditioning and irrational fears.

For example

At the age of 11 I was walking to school with a friend and I ran across the road to join some other friends. I did this without looking and was hit and seriously injured by an oncoming car. I had no recollection of this and was unconscious for a time. However my friend who had witnessed a terrible accident was terrified of crossing roads afterwards. She would stand at the side of the road and not be able to cross over. She had been classically conditioned to not cross the road by having an earlier fearful experience. It would be a phobia as it was irrational and interfered with her normal life because if you take care all roads are safe to cross at some point.

Similarly if a child has been stung by a wasp it may become really scared of wasps and the fear of being stung again may mean the child will not go into the garden and as an adult will always be very fearful of wasps.

Quite a few adults have phobias about birds or spiders; these usually originate from an early unpleasant experience but remain with them and are immediately invoked in the presence of the feared object.

John Watson (1878–1958) will always be associated with his 'Little Albert' *classical conditioning* experiment. Albert was introduced to several different animals. But each time Albert was introduced to a rat a loud noise would be made which frightened Albert. So thereafter every time he saw the rat he was scared, he had been *classically conditioned* to behave in a certain way as an automatic response. Much of Watson's work studying human behaviour has since been discredited and his 'experiments' using children and some of his other ideas would now be considered cruel and unethical. It could also be argued that the behaviourist theory is a study of behaviour and managing behaviours rather than a theory of development.

Burrhus Skinner (1904–90) proposed that reward and punishment were important in strengthening and weakening behaviour. This is referred to as *operant conditioning*. If we are rewarded when performing behaviour we are likely to repeat the behaviour, if we are punished we will avoid the behaviour, although there is unpredictability about this idea. If punishment is stopped when we perform behaviour we are more likely to reproduce the behaviour. He 'taught' animals and birds to do things through 'selective reinforcement' and that positive reinforcement makes children repeat the behaviour whilst negative reinforcement may also result in repeating the behaviour in order to stop something happening. Reinforcement encourages a given behaviour, whether the experience is of positive or negative reinforcement. Actions lead to rewards and consequences. Operant conditioning is used to modify animal behaviour where desirable behaviour is rewarded with a treat as a positive reinforcement thereby increasing the desired behaviour. Skinner's theories are also evident today in behavioural modification and parenting programmes, including the Solihull Approach and Triple P.

Activity

Can you think of some examples of positive reinforcement used by adults towards young children?

For example

Children may be rewarded for good behaviour or completing a task, so behaviour is strengthened, increased or reinforced by a reward. Similarly negative behaviours can be decreased; so behaving badly at school means no school trip. Therefore behaving badly means the withdrawal of something favourable, good behaviour invites a reward.

The difference between Watson's *classical conditioning* and Skinner's *operant conditioning* is that the former involves making an association between an involuntary response and a stimulus. Operant conditioning is about making an association between a voluntary behaviour and a consequence. With operant conditioning the learner is rewarded with incentives, and is an active participant, performing an action in order to be rewarded or punished. Whereas classical conditioning offers no incentives and the learner is passive.

SOCIAL LEARNING THEORY

Albert Bandura is a Canadian psychologist (born 1925). Bandura developed social learning theory, which proposed that children learn by observing others and that observational learning can also occur without reinforcement. He felt that children do not simply respond to stimuli; but rather they interpret stimuli. Children relate by interacting with and learning from people who have meaning and value. He famously demonstrated his theory in 1961 using the 'Bobo doll' experiment (Tassoni et al., 2008).

In families and wider societal contexts children are influenced on multiple levels, including media characters, 'super-heroes' and gender-based influences often being imitated. The responses of others around the child to the behaviour serve as reinforcers which are either negative or positive but will result in changed behaviour (McLeod, 2011).

COGNITIVE THEORIES

Jean Piaget (1896–1980) proposed stages of cognitive development and developed his theory through observation of children. He developed experiential studies designed to test his hypothesis that children develop similar ways of understanding the world at different stages, and that each stage cannot be explained simply in terms of acquiring more knowledge. Piaget's theory was considered radical at the time and challenged behaviourist ideas that children start as a blank slate to be filled in with adult knowledge.

Piaget first trained as a biologist and suggested that humans, like animals, are genetically predisposed (*nature*) to live and behave in certain ways. He became interested in psychology and psychoanalysis and began to think that biology might help to explain psychological development. He proposed that intelligence is to do with making an appropriate *adaption* and that ultimately an *adaption* is a survival mechanism.

He suggested that children develop their understanding of the world through grouping a series of actions with an idea; which he referred to as a *schema*. Simply, a *schema* is a way of organising and making sense of the world. He called these *processes of adaption*:

- *Assimilation:* information and experience may be built upon into an existing schema.
- *Accommodation:* a new schema is created when new experiences don't fit into those that already exist.
- *Equilibration:* these processes are driven by a need to understand the world and discomfort when things don't fit. Schemas may be abandoned altogether and replaced with ones which can encompass new information; in this way the changes can be viewed as qualitative rather than quantitative.

Schemas develop by assimilation, by fitting new structures into old schemas; infant sucking behaviour is a schema. The infant is hungry and experiences disequilibration (instability), so as a consequence demands food and cries.

The care giver or mother responds by feeding the infant, who then achieves *equilibration* (stability).

Growth requires more than milk to sustain development, so weaning is introduced. The infant will need to accommodate this new experience and will develop the old sucking *schema* into a new sucking *schema* using a spoon. Piaget called this process *assimilation* (so fitting the world into existing schemas). Therefore Piaget believed that in achieving new abilities the baby's development is secured and a normal child will quickly develop new schemas, spoons, feeder cups and so on in order to achieve *equilibration*.

Piaget identified four stages of intellectual development:

1. *Sensory motor period (birth–2 years):* alternative ways of achieving the same consequence are discovered (12–18 months).

   Object permanence ... the opposite of 'out of sight out of mind'. Ego-centric ... relating to the world only from own perspective.

2. *Pre-operations period (2–7 years):* developing abilities to use language, symbols and gestures to represent objects, ideas and experience. Child's imagination expands and from 4 onwards speech may be more social although tends to remain egocentric.

   o *Animism:* simple logical concepts.
   o *Moral realism:* rules are inflexible.

3. *Concrete operations stage (7–11 years):* thinking becomes increasingly logical and rational and things may not be as they first appear.

   o *Conservation:* quantity remains the same even when appearance changes.
   o *Reversibility:* physical and mental operations can be reversed.

4. *Formal operations stage (11–16 years):* adolescents learn to think logically about abstract ideas and hypothetical situations (Bee and Boyd, 2010: 143).

Lev Vygotsky (1896–1934) was a Russian psychologist who was mainly interested in children's acquisition of knowledge. His work only became more widely accessible outside Russia from the early 1960s. Similarly to Piaget, he believed that children are active participants in their cognitive development. Although, unlike Piaget, Vygotsky viewed social interaction and context as being intrinsic factors, with cultural influences adding further dimensions which the child would not achieve in isolation. He attempted to create a theory taking into account the interaction between all factors, with the belief that we can only be understood within our social and historical contexts. Vygotsky proposed that development follows a pattern. We initially acquire knowledge and skills through the interpersonal interactions with parents, siblings, other relatives, peers and teachers. The interactions tend to be dynamic and adjusted according to a child's ability. In the context of a 'teacher' and child this would be working just outside a child's ability to manage a task on their own but within a child's ability to manage with help. Vygotsky called this the '*zone of proximal development*'. The difference between Piaget and Vygotsky was that Vygotsky felt that logical thinking emerged as a result of internalising speech patterns and routines from peers and adults rather than schemas constructed through interaction with the physical world as Piaget thought.

Jerome Brunner (born 1915) further developed Vygotsky's theories and introduced the concept of a *spiral curriculum*. This explained that by building on previous knowledge and experience through the help of others, developmental tasks could be accomplished. Ideas and activities would be revisited but used in a different way because of developing cognitive abilities.

Brunner also developed the concept of *scaffolding*. This can be thought about as adults, peers or siblings supporting children to develop and learn in the same way as scaffolding is an essential part of the construction process on a building site. Once the child can support him or herself then the scaffolding (adult support) can be removed.

ECOLOGICAL SYSTEMS THEORY

Urie Bronfenbrenner (1917–2005) was a developmental psychologist who believed that cultural influences are filtered through the family. The family helps to reinforce cultural expectations but can also protect against what might be viewed as negative or harmful influences. Bronfenbrenner co-founded the Head Start programme in the USA in the 1960s which continues today with the addition of Early Head Start. The programme is aimed at supporting low-income families and children from 0 to 5 years. It promotes healthy prenatal outcomes, healthy families and infant and toddler development. The Sure Start programme in Britain started in 1998 and is based on a similar philosophy to the Head Start programmes in the USA. Bronfenbrenner's (1979, 1992 [1989]) theories demonstrated the relationship between environmental influences and how these impact on child development. His principle was that development was a joint function of the person and the environment and continued throughout the life course.

Bronfenbrenner identified three levels or structures:

1. *Micro/mesosystem:* the micro/mesosystem is a pattern of activities, roles and interpersonal relations experienced by the developing person in a given face-to-face setting with particular physical and material features (e.g. home, school and work). The micro/mesosystem also contains other persons with distinctive characteristics of temperament, personality and systems of belief.
2. *Exosystem:* the exosystem encompasses the linkage and processes taking place between two or more settings, at least one of which does not ordinarily contain the developing person, but in which events occur that influence processes within the immediate setting that does contain that person (e.g. for a child, the relation between the home and the parent's workplace; for a parent, the relation between the school and the neighbourhood group). Exosystem elements affect other parts of the microsystem. The effect can be indirect but the influence exists, e.g. parents' work, parents' friends and colleagues. Another example sitting within the exosystem and directly influencing micro/mesosystems is the planned introduction by September 2014 of universal free school meals for infant age children (years 1 and 2) in England. This is an important social policy of which one aspect will result in the free school meals provision and accompanying potential stigma for poor children in this age group disappearing for two years. Just using one aspect from that example; you can understand how changes taking place in the exosystem directly influence a child's micro/mesosystem.
3. *Macrosystem:* the macrosystem consists of the overarching pattern of micro- and exosystems. It encompasses the characteristics of a given culture, subculture or other broader social context, with particular reference to the developmentally instigative belief systems, resources, hazards, lifestyles, opportunity structures, life course options and patterns of social interchange that are embedded in each of these systems. This would include wider systems such as neighbourhoods, the media, culture, ethnicity and social class, where values and ideology are transmitted. The macrosystem may be thought of as a societal blueprint for a particular culture, subculture or other broader social context.

Bronfenbrenner suggested another way of thinking of this by using a Russian doll. The baby nests within many layers or structures of other 'dolls' having direct influence on it and each other. No one exists independently of the other's influence but rather there is continual and ongoing interaction between layers and structures. Similarly Hilary Clinton (2006) stated: '*It takes a village to create a child*'. It is a reminder of Winnicott's statement '*there's no such thing as an infant*' as discussed earlier. Bronfenbrenner's model seeks to demonstrate how individuals relate to the environment and how cultural values and norms become played out in relationships. Movement between the levels involves a change of role for the individual (Beckett and Taylor, 2010: 164).

Activity

Draw Bronfenbrenner's diagram (Figure 2.1) and identify your own micro/meso-, exo- and macrosystems.

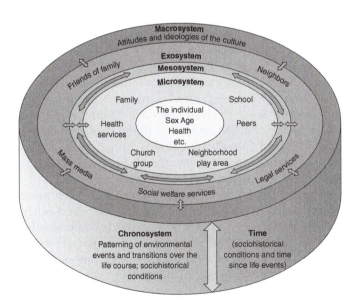

Figure 2.1 Bronfenbrenner's ecological systems model

Source: DH (2013: 124)

Following on from Bronfenbrenner's ecological systems theory it feels useful at this point to take a closer look at influences on family, parenting, culture and thus child development, bearing in mind his systems model of thinking about human development. Perhaps we can bear in mind what Bronfenbrenner said:

> ... in order to develop normally; a child requires progressively more complex joint activity with one or more adults who have an irrational emotional relationship with the child. Somebody's got to be crazy about that kid. That's number one. First, last and always. (National Scientific Council on the Developing Child, 2004a: 1)

THE 'FAMILY' AND PARENTING INFLUENCES ON DEVELOPMENT

'Family' is globally considered to be the natural fundamental unit of society. There is a basic assumption that the family is the natural environment for the growth and wellbeing of its members, especially more vulnerable members such as children and the elderly. Family privacy and autonomy are universally valued throughout societies. The right to a private and family life is guaranteed in human rights law.

According to Hulbert (2003) parents now consider formal training as a more reliable indicator of expertise than hands-on experience. From the beginning of the 20th century magazine articles and books on child rearing began to appear, based on the theorists such as Freud and 'experts' of their respective times: John Watson and Benjamin Spock. Watson's influence and behavioural training approaches have been far reaching. Spock however was influenced by Freud and published the *Common Sense Book of Baby and Child Care*. A revised ninth edition has recently been published, with 50 million copies since the original publication having been sold (Needleman, 2012). Spock took psychoanalytic ideas into the home and introduced to parents the idea that they knew more than they actually thought they did. At the time Spock was seen as radical but nevertheless a welcome alternative to the behaviourist approaches. Each appealed to different sorts of parents; those who favoured strict routines and others with a more relaxed view of bringing up baby. These 'experts' became hugely influential on child rearing techniques and the way parents continue to parent today. Media and TV cannot now be ignored either, with popular programmes such as *Supernanny*. This is further demonstrated by social networking sites such as Mumsnet and Facebook. These have impacted greatly on parenting styles and are not always without controversy. Parenting styles are considered to be important influences on child development and outcomes. Baumrind (1991) classified four parenting styles: authoritarian, permissive, uninvolved and authoritative.

It is generally considered that an *authoritative* style of parenting acts as a protective factor, and is the most predicative of positive child outcomes. Authoritative parenting is combines warmth and an affectionate bond of attachment being built between the child and the primary care giver from infancy. It is about a combination of warmth, reasoning, responsiveness, firm limit setting and parental involvement in learning (Huang and Isaacs, 2007).

Activity

Consider your own parenting style (if you are a parent, or what it might be if you became a parent or how were you parented as a child), how does this differ to your parents and grandparents, why do you think this is?

AGE-RELATED STAGES OF CHILD DEVELOPMENT AND ACCOMPANYING THEORIES

Infancy (0–5)

It is important to consider pregnancy as a developmental phase. A 'foetus' is the terminology which describes the organism from about the first 8 weeks of life until birth at about 40 weeks' gestation; literally translated as meaning 'young one' (Music, 2011). Reflexes are present by the fifth month with eyes that can open and close by the sixth month. At 22–26 weeks the 'age of viability' is deemed reached so the foetus is sufficiently developed to survive if born prematurely. Already before the baby is born he or she is subject to the interaction between nature and nurture and is being exposed to his or her environment and socialisation. Studies have shown babies expressing preferences for Dr Seuss stories heard in the womb (DeCasper and Spence, 1986, cited in Music, 2011: 27).

The environment can be a risky place for the developing child, depending on what mother and baby are exposed to. For example teratogens cause birth defects and include chemicals, medications and infections or other diseases in the mother. Thalidomide was a drug taken by expectant mothers in the 1960s to help with morning sickness. Sadly many babies were born from these mothers with deformed limbs or limbs missing. Other examples of teratogens include alcohol, cigarettes and prescription and illegal drugs or diseases the mother may be exposed to and experience such as Rubella. Other environmental risks include maternal stress where there are higher levels of cortisol crossing the placenta. This has the potential to alter the infant's capacity for regulation. The effect of prenatal stress, which affects all psychological systems including attachment, can extend into childhood and adulthood (Lange, 2012). The recent study 'September 11, 2001 Mothers, Infants and Young Children Project' followed the unborn infants of mothers and theorised a risk of 'dyadic trauma'. It is thought that not only the traumatic event in itself has an impact, but perhaps of even greater significance is the parental response to trauma and how this affects the mother–infant dyad in a relational context (Markese, 2012). The project also identified that the unborn infants of these mothers showed altered cortisol levels at one year of age (Yehuda et al., 2005 in Beebe and Jaffa, 2012: 13).

The way birth is experienced varies hugely. Life expectancy is dependent on where we are born. In some areas of the developing world child mortality is high, as it has been in the UK in previous centuries. But even today in Britain a postcode can determine how long you might live. A World Health Organisation study in 2008, later known as the 'Glasgow Effect' showed an example of stark health inequities, noting that a boy in a deprived Glasgow area had an average life expectancy of 54 years compared with a boy from an affluent area 12 km away, with a life expectancy of 82 years (Reid, 2011).

Birth complications can lead to medical interventions such as assisted deliveries and Caesarean sections. Caesarean births can double the infant and mother's complications including risk of infection, longer hospitalisation and increased risk of respiratory problems and reduced short-term responsiveness.

Early emotional experiences are embedded in the architecture of the brains of young children as a response to individual relational experiences and environmental influences. These develop at the same time as mobility (motor skills), thinking (cognition) and communication (language) (National Scientific Council on the Developing Child, 2004b). Neuroscience further demonstrates that the accelerated growth spurts of the brain begin in the last few weeks of pregnancy, continuing until 18–24 months of age. Babies' brains develop with another important person in their life. A reminder of Winnicott's statement that there is no such thing as an infant without a mother. Optimal attachment relationships are essential as they facilitate the self-regulatory mechanism in the brain. The infant's primary goal in the first year of life is to establish attachment of emotional communication and to develop self-regulation (Schore, 2005). The quality of care impacts greatly, if feelings are unmanaged thinking is impaired, but if there are positive early relationships cognitive development is improved.

Activity

Have a look at the following observation and consider relevant child development theory. When thinking about applying theory it is a good idea to always think about the context, remember: 'there is no such thing as a baby ...'. You will see several theories have been applied. If you were however conducting an observation it is best to consider and develop one or two theories at length rather than a 'throwing everything at it' approach which is seen here.

Background

Elsie is 2 years and 5 months old. She has a brother 'John' who is 5 months old. Elsie has parents, mum and dad, and they all share the same household. Elsie's dad works long hours on weekdays so Elsie is mainly looked after by her mum when both parents are not together. They live in a house where Elsie has her own bedroom. Elsie enjoys preschool in the village where she goes one morning per week. She sees a lot of her wider family every week, including both sets of grandparents, uncles, aunts and cousins.

Observation

Grandmother is visiting and asks Elsie if they can go out to the garden to see the veg patch. Elsie says 'let's go', she is very excited. 'Hang on a minute let's put your pants, leggings, socks and wellies on!' Grandmother helps Elsie to dress and comments on the pants with spots on (Elsie is in her first week of potty training, hence no nappy on). There is a sticker chart on the wall with at least 40 stickers in the 'wee' section and about 10 stickers in the 'poo' section.

Grandmother finishes helping Elsie with her wellies, they open the back door and go out into the garden holding hands.

'Wow!' says grandmother when they get to the veg patch, which is a square that has been dug out with the soil turned over looking ready for planting. There is a path of stepping stones. 'You can cross over by walking on these', says Elsie, pointing where grandmother should cross, which she does, all the way over and back again while Elsie watches. Grandmother suggests Elsie has a go. Elsie starts to cross over the stones raising her arms up exactly as grandmother has done while trying to balance. Carefully she steps over each stone and then gets to the last one, there is quite a gap between the edge of the stone and the grass beyond the patch. 'Go on you can jump', grandmother suggests. 'No', Elsie says in a daring sort of way as if it could be dangerous. 'OK I will help you.' So grandmother steps onto the stones behind Elsie and taking her hands helps her jump off onto the grass.

Suggested application of theories

Bowlby: Attachment: demonstrates secure attachment to a secondary attachment figure (grandparent).

Brunner: Scaffolding theory: support to complete a task which can then be accomplished on one's own.

Piaget (cognitive): Sensory motor period (birth–2 years) also the pre-operations period (2–7 years).

Erikson: Second stage of Erikson's eight stages of development: autonomy vs shame and doubt (developing a sense of independence).

Freud: 1–3 years anal stage: pleasure becomes focused around elimination. Conflict may emerge as a result of the parent's attempts to toilet train.

Bion: Experience and containment.

Skinner: Operant conditioning – the star chart.

Vygotsky: The zone of proximal development: social interaction and context considered as crucial.

Bandura: Observational learning – copying grandmother when stepping onto stones.

Bronfenbrenner: Ecological systems: family, dad's job, preschool and their community, micro/meso- exo- and macrosystems.

Childhood (5–11)

The childhood years continue with ongoing brain development and physical growth spurts. There is a meeting of neurological, physical, cognitive and socioemotional development. Children in Britain will have started full-time school in the year of their fourth birthday. So for some children they may only just be 4 and for others they may be nearly 5 depending on their birth date. Going to school is a huge transition point in a child's life – separating from care givers, parents and family for several hours a day and experiencing a new environment and relationships, with the accompanying routines and expectations.

Activity

Have a look at the following observation and apply relevant child development theory.

Joe is 7 and in a primary school class with 20 other boys and girls. The classroom is sunny and bright with equipment, book shelves and storage boxes all around the room. There are posters and picture on the walls. The teacher has a whiteboard. All the children sit at tables which are joined up in groups. So there are four children to each group of tables. They are facing each other and not the teacher, who is standing at the front of the class. There is a teaching assistant helping Joe with his task. Joe has a diagnosis of ADHD so he is easily distracted and finds it difficult to concentrate for very long and is sometimes impulsive.

Joe is colouring in letter shapes and then cutting them out to stick on a poster. While he is colouring he keeps looking around the classroom and shouts over to his friend on another table who waves back. Joe starts talking to the boy opposite him. The other children round the table are busy working and cutting out. He is trying to concentrate but finds it difficult to stay on task. The teaching assistant reminds Joe to keep on colouring and then she helps him with the scissors and cutting out a letter R. Joe manages to cut out a letter L for which he receives praise. At the end of the lesson Joe receives a gold star for working hard. He rushes outside at break and tears round the playground with the other boys.

Suggested theories applied

Freud: Joe is in the latency stage (5–puberty) where his focus is now on developing social and intellectual skills. It is a relatively 'latent' or quiet period prior to entering the genital phase of adolescence. During these years peer relationships are primarily with those of the same gender.

Erikson: Similarly to Freud's latency stage, Joe is Erikson's industry vs inferiority stage (6–adolescence), where he is learning intellectual and social skills.

Piaget: During the concrete operations stage (7–11) the child starts to be able to think logically and have a better understanding of mental operations. For example bananas belong to the group 'fruit' and that Joe's pet dog Jim is a Jack Russell, a Jack Russell is a dog and that a dog is an animal.

Bowlby: Attachment theory: teachers and teaching assistants can represent significant secondary attachment figures. There is not enough information to summarise Joe's attachment quality but the observation does demonstrate a capacity to make use of support, which may mean he has a secure type of attachment quality as this is what his earlier experiences may have been; one of support from primary care givers. He also seems to have positive peer relationships.

Skinner: Operant conditioning: the use of a reward system, the gold star.

Bandura: Observational learning: Joe is trying to stay on task as the other boys are.

Vygotsky: The interaction between the teaching assistant and Joe is what Vygotsky called the zone of proximal development. He is being supported to complete a task just outside his ability until he can manage on his own.

Brunner: Scaffolding theory: Joe is being supported by the teaching assistant to complete a task until he can manage by himself.

Bronfenbrenner: The system around Joe, here it is school, is also instrumental in supporting his development and would be a part of Joe's micro/mesosystem. Additionally, school is also influenced by education policy, both locally and centrally, therefore positioned in Joe's exosystem.

It also has to be borne in mind Joe has a diagnosis of ADHD so has problems in the areas of concentration, hyperactivity and impulsivity (the triad of impairments). There may be potential significant difficulties for Joe to negotiate in addition to the developmental tasks or 'milestones' expected of him. For a child like Joe a busy classroom can be a challenging environment.

Adolescence (11–18)

Anna Freud aptly described the adolescent phase as follows:

> It is normal for an adolescent to behave for a considerable length of time in an inconsistent and unpredictable manner; to fight his impulses to accept them; to ward them off successfully and to be overrun by them; to love his parents and to hate them; to revolt against them and to be deeply dependent upon them; to be deeply ashamed to acknowledge his mother before others and unexpectedly to desire heart to heart talks with her; to thrive on imitation of and identification with others while searching unceasingly for his own identity; to be more idealistic, artistic, generous and unselfish than he will ever be again but also the opposite: self centred, egotistic, calculating. Such fluctuations would be deemed highly abnormal at any other time of life. (Freud, 1958: 255–8)

The only other time in life where such rapid changes, initiated by the hypothalamus, occur is in the womb. The rapidity of change brings about enormous psychological upheaval and physical changes including development of sexual characteristics, not always coinciding with emotional states of mind. Adolescence is a complex adjustment, on the child's part, to major physical and emotional changes and is a highly important developmental process (Waddell, 2002: 139). Of course continuing to 'build a brain' in adolescence does not develop in isolation of a parallel biological process that is triggered by hormonal activity. This in itself has an enormous effect in terms of psychological upheaval.

There are three major growth spurts in brain and nervous system development. Between 10 and 12 there is a major increase in neurons in the frontal cortex (thinking, reasoning, logic and decision making). An excess of connections and synapses grow with many becoming pruned, leaving the remaining connections to develop. Between 13 and 15, spatial and motor functions include qualitative changes in nerve pathways enabling abstract thinking. From 17 years onwards changes in the frontal lobes enable increased ability for planning and logical thinking. The amygdala, responsible for emotional regulation, is highly active during adolescence and tends to dominate often leading to misunderstanding and conflict (Morgan, 2013).

There will also be a growth spurt in size: adolescents may grow by up to 15 cm per year. Peak age of growth in girls is between 12 and 13 and for boys 15 and 16. Puberty comprises a number of milestones which result in the ability to reproduce. Other developments include an increase in memory capacity, and a developing awareness of mental processes, techniques and strategies.

Early adolescence (12–16) is characterised by major changes in every aspect of development and functioning. Late adolescence (16–20) is a time when changes are consolidated and individual identity is established.

As Briggs (2002: 12) observes: 'The search for identity takes place in a psychosocial matrix, forced upon the adolescent by the impact of puberty from within and the social contexts, demands and rituals from the outside.'

Briggs (2002: 12) further suggests a young person has to consider: 'who am I and who am I like? And also who am I not?'

Identity formation can be an increasingly complex task in relation to different relationships and cultural influences. Ethnic identity formation in adolescence involves social and internal processes. For the ethnic minority adolescent this can be a difficult, exacting process of developing cohesiveness, and a sense of self within divisive and complex contexts. There are pressures on ethnic minority adolescents to assimilate to another culture which may have quite differing characteristics and values. Sorting 'me' from the 'not me', being able to differentiate sameness and difference are at the fore of adolescent experiences.

Understanding about sex roles may increase anxiety and becomes a central issue with regard to identity. There is a shift from same sex friendships to mixed sex relationships. In later adolescence friends increasingly become sources of emotional and social support. Theories about cognitive development at this stage can be applied to ideas about developing social relationships (Rubin et al., 2005, cited in Bee and Boyd, 2010: 313). However, there are unique characteristics. Social interaction requires understanding of social rules and expectations of how people are likely to behave and react. Peer groups, cliques (same sex), crowds (stereotyped groups) become more evident and numbers increase; friendships become more intense; family relationships undergo change.

Activity

Have a look at the following observation and consider relevant child development theory.

> Lisa is 16. She is attending an initial Tier 3 CAMHS (Child and Adolescent Mental Health Services) appointment following a referral from her GP over concerns about self-harm (cutting). She had also taken an overdose of a small amount of paracetamol. Lisa attends with her mum who she seems to have a warm relationship with. The family are from the Traveller community living in settled housing.
>
> Lisa presents as being unhappy although she is able to engage in conversation and tells her story of moving around three different primary schools and was now at her third secondary school, all local to her home. The reason for the moves had been over poor behaviour and Lisa reported getting into trouble quite a lot. Lisa says she has a boyfriend and is tearful when mum states she does not want Lisa to see him any more as he has been abusive towards Lisa. Lisa talks favourably about her other peers. At one point she looks at the clock in the room and tells me she cannot tell the time, neither can she read beyond a minimal level.

Suggested theories applied

Freud: Genital stage (begins in puberty and continues throughout life): Lisa has developed a sexual relationship with a peer.

Erikson: Identity vs identity diffusion (adolescence–20 years): Lisa is wrestling with her identity in terms of the past with her family and new relationships with peers.

Piaget: Formal operations stage (11–16): although Lisa fits this stage in relation to her chronological age clearly there are some tasks (telling the time and reading) she has not attained. Her intellectual development may be considered impaired and in terms of cognitive skills she has possibly not met her developmental milestones, although she may be intellectually very able.

Bronfenbrenner: Ecological systems theory: Lisa's micro/meso-, macro- and exosystems will consist of her family, a variety of schools, and other relationships. Also included in the macrosystem would be belief systems, and Traveller ethnicity and culture in relation not only to her own values but those of the wider majority culture and how these interact with each other.

Bowlby: Attachment: Lisa enjoys a positive relationship with mum which may indicate secure attachment potentially acting as a protective factor as we do not know much about their earlier relationship.

You will have noticed theoretical similarities with the above cases between Freud and Erikson. In the latter two child and adolescent cases Joe has ADHD and Lisa is exhibiting some concerning behaviours indicative of emotional distress. Young people like Joe and Lisa face potential further difficulties in their development with potential life-long implications given their additional problems. Developmental theory does not take these anomalies into account as theories tend to focus on 'normal developmental' expectations.

Adolescence is often a time of turbulence and risks and hazards to which adolescents are exposed. This can lead to vulnerability in developing psychosocial disorders which peak during adolescence. These include suicide, self-harm, substance misuse, offending behaviour, depression and eating disorders.

CONCLUSION

Attachment theory is probably the most important and relevant theory today and is reaffirmed by neuroscience research as taking precedence over cognitive development. Affect regulation determines the architecture of the brain and is laid down within a context of a nurturing, sensitive hierarchy of attachment relationships. Bronfenbrenner's ecological systems model further demonstrates immediate and wider environmental influences. There are important implications for educationalists where there is an ever increasing focus on learning often at the expense of supporting emotional and social learning. Supporting children, young people, parents, families and communities in nurturing and tending to relationships is a priority for optimal emotional development.

REFERENCES

Anna Freud Centre (2013) The Anna Freud Centre. Available from: www.annafreud.org/pages/history.html (accessed July 2013).

Barrows, P. (2004) Fathers and Families: Locating the Ghost in the Nursery. *Infant Mental Health Journal*, 25 (5): 408–23.

Baumrind, D. (1991) The Influence of Parenting Style on Adolescent Competence and Substance Use. *Journal of Early Adolescence*, 11 (1): 56–95.

Beckett, C. and Taylor, H. (2010) *Human Growth and Development*, 2nd edn. London: Sage.

Bee, H. and Boyd, D. (2010) *The Developing Child*, 12th edn. Boston, MA: Pearson Education.

Beebe, B. and Jaffe, J. (2012) Description of the Project: A Longitudinal Primary Prevention Project for Mothers Pregnant and Widowed in the World Trade Center Tragedy of September 11, 2001, and their Young Children. In Beebe, B., Cohen, P., Sossin, K.M. and Markese, S. (eds), *Infants and Young Children of September 11, 2001: A Primary Intervention Project*. London and New York: Routledge.

Bowlby, J. (1952) *Maternal Care and Mental Health*. Geneva: World Health Organization.

Bowlby, J. (1988) *A Secure Base*. London: Routledge.

Briggs, S. (2002) *Working with Adolescents: A Contemporary Psychodynamic Approach*. Basingstoke: Palgrave Macmillan.

Bronfenbrenner, U. (1979) *The Ecology of Human Development*. Cambridge, MA: Harvard University Press.

Bronfenbrenner, U. (1992 [1989]) Ecological Systems Theory. In Vasta, R. (ed.) *Six Theories of Child Development, Revised Formulations and Current Issues*. London: Jessica Kingsley, pp. 187–250.

Calabrese, M.L., Farber, B.A. and Westen, D. (2005) The Relationship of Adult Attachment Constructs to Object Relational Patterns of Representing Self and Others. *Journal of the American Academy of Psychoanalysis and Dynamic Psychiatry*, 33 (3): 513–30.

Department of Health (2013) *CMO Report: Our Children Deserve Better: Prevention Pays*. London: DH.

Diem-Wille, G. (2011) *The Early Years of Life Psychoanalytic Development Theory According to Freud, Klein and Bion*. London: Karnac.

Douglas, H. (2007) *Containment and Reciprocity: Integrating Psychoanalytic Theory and Child Development Research for Work with Children*. Hove: Routledge.

Freud, A. (1958) Adolescence. *Psychoanalytic Study of the Child*, 13: 255–78. Available from: www.beyondthecouch.org/0307/anna_freud_quotes_0307.htm (accessed July 2013).

Gerhardt, S. (2004) *Why Love Matters; How Affection Shapes a Baby's Brain*. Hove: Brunner Routledge.

Gibson, M. (2006) *Order from Chaos Responding to Traumatic Incidents*, 3rd edn. Bristol: The Policy Press.

Goldberg, S., Muir, R. and Kerr, J. (2000) *Attachment Theory: Social, Developmental, and Clinical Perspectives*. London: Routledge.

Howe, D. (2011) *Attachment across the Lifecourse: A Brief Introduction*. Basingstoke: Palgrave Macmillan.

Huang, I.N. and Isaacs, M.R. (2007) Early Childhood Mental Health: A Focus on Culture and Context. In Perry, D., Kaufmann, R. and Knitzer, J. (eds) *Social and Emotional Health in Early Childhood*. Baltimore and London: Brookes Publishing Co., pp. 37–59.

Hulbert, A. (2003) *Raising America: Experts, Parents and a Century of Advice about Children*. New York: Alfred Knopf.

Lange, A. (2012) Prenatal Maternal Stress and the Developing Fetus and Infant: A Review of Animal Models as Related to Human Research. In Beebe, B., Cohen, P., Sossin, K.M. and Markese, S. (eds) *Mothers, Infants and Young Children of September 11, 2001: A Primary Prevention Project*. London and New York: Routledge, pp. 175–89.

Lindon, J. (2010) *Understanding Child Development: Linking Theory and Practice*, 2nd edn. London: Hodder Education.

McLeod, S.A. (2011) *Albert Bandura: Social Learning Theory, Simply Psychology*. Available from: www.simplypsychology.org/bandura.html (accessed July 2013).

Markese, S. (2012) Dyadic Trauma in Infancy and Early Childhood: Review of the Literature. In Beebe, B., Cohen, P., Sossin, K.M. and Markese, S. (eds) *Mothers, Infants and Young Children of September 11, 2001: A Primary Intervention Project*. London and New York: Routledge, pp. 190–227.

Mawson, C. (2012) *Furthering the Psychoanalytic Theory and Technique of Melanie Klein. Wilfred Bion*. The Melanie Klein Trust. Available from: www.melanie-klein-trust.org.uk/?location_id=17 (accessed July 2013).

Morgan, N. (2013) *Blame My Brain: The Amazing Teenage Brain Revealed*. London: Walker Books.

Music, G. (2011) *Nurturing Natures Attachment and Children's Sociocultural and Brain Development*. Hove: Psychology Press.

National Scientific Council on the Developing Child (2004a) *Young Children Develop in an Environment of Relationships*, Working Paper No. 1. Center on the Developing

Child, Harvard University, USA. Available from: www.developingchild.net (accessed July 2013).

National Scientific Council on the Developing Child (2004b) *Children's Emotional Development is Built into the Architecture of Their Brains*, Working Paper No. 2, Center on the Developing Child, Harvard University, USA. Available from: www.developingchild. net (accessed July 2013).

Needleman, R. (2012) *Dr. Spock's Baby and Childcare*, 9th edn. New York and London: Simon & Schuster.

Reid, M. (2011) Behind the Glasgow Effect. *Bulletin of the World Health Organization*, 89 (10): 701–76. Available from: www.who.int/bulletin/volumes/89/10/11-021011/en/index. html, (accessed July 2013).

Reiss, D. (1998) Mechanisms Linking Genetic and Social Influences in Adolescent Development: Beginning a Collaborative Search. *Current Directions in Psychological Science*, 6: 100–5.

Rutter, M. (2002) Nature, Nurture, and Development: From Evangelism through Science toward Policy and Practice. *Child Development,* 73 (1): 1–21.

Schore, A. (2005) Attachment, Affect Regulation and the Developing Right Brain: Linking Development Neuroscience to Pediatrics. *Pediatrics in Review*, 26 (6): 204–211. Available at: www.allanschore.com/pdf/__SchorePediatricsInReview.pdf (accessed November 2013).

Spelke, E. (1991) Physical Knowledge in Infancy: Reflections on Piaget's Theory. In Carey, S. and Gelman, R. (eds) *The Epeigenesis of Mind: Essays on Biology and Cognition*. Mahwah, NJ: Lawrence Erlbaum, pp. 133–69.

Tassoni, P., Bulman, K. and Beith, K. (2008) *Children's Care Learning and Development*. Harlow: Heinemann.

Waddell, M. (2002) *Inside Lives Pschoanalysis and the Growth of the Personality*. London: Karnac.

Winnicott, D.W. (1956) Primary Maternal Preoccupation. *Through Paediatrics to Psychoanalysis*. London: Hogarth Press and the Institute of Psychoanalysis, pp. 300–5.

Winnicott, D.W. (2012) *Deprivation and Delinquency*, ed. Winnicott, C., Shepherd, R. and Davis, M. London: Routledge.

3

SAFEGUARDING CHILDREN AND YOUNG PEOPLE AND CHILDREN'S RIGHTS

MADDIE BURTON

Overview

- Historical overview
  - Early days, later days and public awareness
- Emerging lessons, legislation and policy
  - High profile cases
- Effects; who is abusing whom and why?
  - The 'toxic trio'
- 'Family', recognising abuse and how to respond; multi and inter-agency approaches
  - Awareness
  - Categories of abuse
- Introduction to children's rights
  - The United Nations Convention on the Rights of the Child (1989)
  - *Every Child Matters* (2003)
- Consent and confidentiality
- Case studies and student/reader activities throughout the chapter

INTRODUCTION

Safeguarding children and young people was aptly described by Lord Laming (2003) in two words within *The Victoria Climbié Inquiry* as 'everybody's responsibility'. Subsequently, following the death of baby Peter Connelly in 2007 Lord Laming was asked to write another report: *The Protection of Children in England: A Progress Report* (2009: 7). In his summing up Lord Laming advised 'NOW JUST DO IT'.

Lord Laming's comments, located within six words, 'everybody's responsibility' and 'now just do it', probably sum up where we hope child protection in England today should be. His inquiry and report highlighted ways of working to protect children. It showed where the inter-agency approach both works and does not always work with, sadly, the worst imaginable outcomes. The high-profile case of Victoria Climbié, the subject of Lord Laming's inquiry, led to the creation of the government policy *Every Child Matters* (DfES, 2003) which underpinned the implementation of the Children Act 2004. Professor Eileen Munro's (2011) review, *The Munro Review of Child Protection: Final Report – A Child Centred System*, is the most recent review with key phrases including '*early* help' and '*child*-centred'.

Though it may feel as though there is an element of 'shock and awe' to this chapter, it is not aimed at sensationalism of any sort. It is a snapshot of the subject. But we cannot underestimate the ongoing seriousness, depth and breadth of child protection and safeguarding today and the implications for children and young people and their mental health and wellbeing. Neither can we underestimate the problems faced in making it our responsibility or ensuring that appropriate action is taken when necessary to safeguard children. We owe it to children and young people to be vigilant about our responses and to ensure our concerns are acted upon.

The chapter will look at safeguarding from a historical and contemporary perspective and consider the process of safeguarding today. What is 'everybody's responsibility' and what does it mean? What are the responsibilities of all workers, professionals, agencies and those coming into contact with children? How should we 'just do it' and act in 'best interest' and place children at the heart of the safeguarding process as Lord Laming urged? Recognising signs of abuse, and direction on how to respond will be explored with be reference to current government policy and legislation. The potentially devastating long-term effects of child abuse, often throughout generations, will be considered and links made with Chapters 1 and 2. Children's rights will also be introduced.

HISTORICAL OVERVIEW

Early days

It is important to acknowledge and understand the historical context of safeguarding. Child and infant mortality has previously been high in Britain. Infants and children died from what are now preventable diseases. In the early 19th century rates were between 50 and 75% for infants up to age 5. By 1900–2 there were 142 deaths per 1000 infants up to age 1. By 2000 that figure had reduced to 5.5 deaths per 1000. This has further reduced to 4.1 in 2011 as a provisional figure at the time of writing (Office for National Statistics, 2011). State immunisation programmes, since the inception of the NHS in 1948, have considerably reduced childhood mortality in the 20th and 21st centuries; although there have been reductions in recent years in the uptake of immunisations, leading to a return of previously virtually eradicated diseases in England such as mumps, measles and whooping cough. Improved nutrition, the provision of school milk, school meals and free school meals for poorer children have all contributed to reductions in childhood mortality. Added to this are overall public health improvements, housing and education, increased safety awareness in homes, travel, roads and the community; for example, fireguards, smoke alarms, fire retardant clothing and upholstery, safety gates, stair gates, seat belts, traffic calming measures in built-up areas and around schools. All of the above government intervention programmes have contributed to a significant reduction in child mortality than was seen in previous centuries. Although it is interesting and concerning to note recent reports of significant numbers of children and families not able to afford enough food and the increasing numbers of 'Food Banks' being set up throughout the UK at the time of writing. The charity Trussell Trust provided emergency food to over 50,000 people, one-third of whom were children, in a four-month period in 2012 (Molly, 2012). Free school meals and extended schools are only available during term time and not in school holidays.

Later days: have we really moved on?

Despite some significant changes in the last and present century there is a feeling we have some way to go before we shake off the attitudes of the past, which still seem to seep into our contemporary lives even though we may not be aware of this. For example up until as late as 1967, a mere 40 or so years ago, children from Britain were being emigrated to the former colonies including North America, Australia, Zimbabwe, South Africa and the Caribbean. This started as long ago as 1618, and during a peak between 1870 and 1914 some 80,000 children were emigrated to Canada in that period alone. The Poor Law Amendment Act 1850 allowed children under 16 to be sent overseas. It is estimated a total number of 150,000 children with an average age of 9.4 and some of the youngest being only 2 were deported. Many children had positive experiences but many did not. It took until 2009 for the Australian government to issue a formal apology, followed by the British government in 2010 (National Archives, 2013).

It feels appropriate at this juncture to remind ourselves of comments made in a UNICEF (2007) report:

> The true measure of a nation's standing is how well it attends to its children: their health and safety, their material security, their education and socialization, and their sense of being loved, valued, and included in the families and societies into which they are born. (UNICEF, 2007: 1)

Would you be surprised to discover that the report, looking at 21 Organisation for Economic Co-operation and Development (OECD) countries and drawing on data from 2001–2003, found the UK is nearly at the bottom of the list in position 20 with the USA at 21? The report looked at infant mortality, material wellbeing, health and safety, educational wellbeing, family and peer relationships, behaviours and risks and subjective wellbeing. The latest child well-being report makes interesting reading and, drawing on data from 2009 and 2010, finds the UK having improved its over-all position by 4 places to 16 out of the 29 countries studied (UNICEF, 2013). It is expected that following the continued economic downturn since the data was collected a less improved picture may be revealed. The report demonstrated that children are less happy in some of the richest countries in the world (Alderson, 2008).

Public awareness

The notion that children could be abused by their parents and care givers was only first posited, again relatively recently, by paediatrician Dr Harold Kempe in 1962 where, with other colleagues in the USA, he first proposed 'non-accidental injury' in a paper entitled 'The Battered Child Syndrome' (Kempe et al., 1985). In defining it as a 'syn-drome' professionals could be seen as the 'experts' in identifying and making a diagnosis. The paper emerged via the National Society for the Prevention of Cruelty to Children (NSPCC) in England shortly afterwards and influenced their approach and that of government policy (Parton, 2006). The NSPCC was founded in 1884. Interestingly, the Cruelty to Animals Act 1829 predated any child protection legisla-tion in the USA and UK. In the latter part of the 1960s the NSPCC took on the role of educating other professional groups outside the medical profession and started to promote child abuse issues in the media and with government. During the 1980s and in 1987, led by the NSPCC and TV presenter Esther Rantzen, helplines including 'ChildLine' were established. In its 25-year history ChildLine have counselled 2.6 million children on issues including bullying, physical and sexual abuse. In keeping with changing times, in 2009 the ChildLine website was launched (NSPCC, 2012).

A feature of many of the publicised cases is often one of systemic failure within the organisations and agencies with the very powers invested in them to protect children. There seems to be an ongoing struggle to find the right balance between too much intervention and too little (Hendry and Macinnes, 2011). Demonstrated again recently in the Rochdale report and Lord Carlile's report into the Edlington case (Carlile, 2012), which will be discussed later in the chapter. The 'integrated approach to safeguarding' often fails children and is evident it is not always working. The unique status of chil-dren and young people mean that virtually all will be in contact with statutory agen-cies such as health and education at some point and often at frequent points during their childhood from pre-birth to adolescence. This indicates there will also be many points of contact with professionals, such as midwives, health visitors, GP's, workers in early year's settings, school staff including teachers, teaching assistants and school nurses. Many of whom will work together within the models of multi and inter-agency working. Everyone with responsibilities for working with children and young people are required to undergo safeguarding training and all have a *responsibility* to do so, together with their employing agencies and organisations. Children and young people are dependent on others not only to notice their plight but to take appropriate action.

With many of the publicised cases it has been found that often it is a member of the public who takes decisive action in terms of safeguarding, despite the children being already known to a variety of professionals and agencies. Kyra Ischak was an eight-year-old girl who died in 2008 from the effects of severe malnutrition despite concerns raised by members of the public and teaching staff at her school (Birmingham Safeguarding Children Board, 2010).

Many of those in contact with children, young people and the public are raising concerns through recognised channels, yet often concerns are not always acted upon appropriately.

EMERGING LESSONS, LEGISLATION AND POLICY FROM HIGH PROFILE CASES

Maria Colwell: the first of the major child abuse inquiries

The death of Maria Colwell in 1973 led to the first major child abuse inquiry. Maria was the youngest of five children. Maria was known to Children's Services and the NSPCC. Maria had been returned to her mother's care after a period of time in family/foster care. On 7 January 1973 Maria was taken in a pram to hospital by her mother and stepfather where she was pronounced dead as a result of internal injuries and severe bruising. Maria's death led to changes in policy and practice and the child care systems we have in place today. By 1976 all areas held registers of children at risk of abuse. Models and ways of working would now include 'case conferences' and 'key workers' (Hobart and Frankel, 2005). By 1980 the criteria of 'abuse' was extended to include not only physical abuse, which until then had been the main focus, but also severe and persistent neglect and emotional abuse.

It is interesting to consider the current media attention on public organisations and public figures concerning sexual abuse allegations. When one views recorded footage of television programmes from the 1970s the behaviour of TV presenters towards the invited children in the studio would be considered unacceptable now. But few raised concerns then, despite the programmes being watched by millions. On reflection perhaps one can see why sexual abuse had not specifically been included before in the Children Act, and then not until the 1989 Act. Until the 1980s sexual abuse was not included unless it was associated with physical injury, and it took until then for it to be included in the child abuse framework for the first time. During the 1980s and 1990s many allegations of sexual abuse emerged from children in residential care settings leading to several inquiries and culminating in a review by Lord Carlile (2002). For the first time child abuse was broadened and relocated outside the family (Parton, 2006). According to recent figures in a research report commissioned by the NSPCC, one in nine young adults (11.3%) experienced contact sexual abuse during childhood. There were 17,727 sexual crimes recorded against children under 16 in England and Wales in 2010/11. It was identified in the report that as a result of abuse there is a strong association between child and adolescent mental health particularly in terms of poorer emotional well-being, self-harm and suicidal thoughts (Radford et al., 2011).

OTHER CASES AND SUBSEQUENT INQUIRIES

Cleveland

Between 1987 and 1988 what became known as the Report of the Inquiry into Child Abuse in Cleveland took place, conducted by Lord Justice Butler-Sloss. The then Health Minister had called for a statutory inquiry following concerns about a number of children in Cleveland being identified as victims of sexual abuse by paediatrician Dr Marietta Higgs, supported by a second consultant paediatrician, Dr Geoffrey Wyatt. The children Dr Higgs saw had attended hospital for other reasons but Dr Higgs had concerns they may have been victims of sexual abuse and admitted the children into hospital straightaway. Initially 10 children were admitted and eventually a total of 125 children were involved over a five-month period. The method she used to determine whether sexual abuse had taken place or not was the 'anal dilation test'. There was also a huge media furore. Dr Higgs' allegations were discredited and 98 of the children returned to their homes and 27 wardship cases were dismissed, with no further proceedings (*British Medical Journal*, 1988). It is interesting to consider that at that time the focus of sexual abuse was about contact abuse and establishing if this had occurred or not. Whereas today, sexual abuse can include a wide range of non-contact and contact abuse. The question of what actually happened to these children remained unresolved but rather the inquiry focused on the way professionals behaved and the way allegations were dealt with (Parton, 2006: 42). The Cleveland Inquiry set out recommendations that:

- The child must be treated as a person not an object of concern;
- The child must not be subjected to 'examinations' or 'disclosure' interviews;
- Professionals must act in 'best interest' at all times;
- No single person or agency should make decisions in isolation;
- More extensive training for professionals was needed;
- Parents should be offered the same courtesy as parents of any referred child.

As a result of Cleveland most of the old law was abolished and was followed by the Children Act 1989. There was a new emphasis on parental responsibility. Parental responsibility was defined as rights and powers that by law a parent or parents have in relation to their child. It is acknowledged that parenting is not only about biological and genetic components but that there are also legal and social aspects (Gardner and Cleaver, 2009). The Act further acknowledged the importance of the child's wishes and that children and young people should be treated as individuals and that both parents and children should be involved through negotiation and in partnership with professionals. Responsibilities of local authorities changed with Section 17 of the Act providing them with a statutory responsibility in relation to children in need (Parton, 2006).

Victoria Climbié

The next decade saw the high-profile case of the death of Victoria Climbié. Victoria arrived in England in 1999. She was sent here by her parents from West Africa to the care of her great aunt, in the hope of a better life. Ten months later in 2000, she died from horrific injuries at the hands of her great aunt (Koauo) and her aunt's boyfriend (Manning). During her short time alive in England she was known to 12 different agencies yet no one spoke to her in her own language (French) or recognised her ill treatment. Wrong assumptions were made, for example, with regard to African culture: that children normally 'stood to attention'. Despite two hospital admissions there was poor inter-agency liaison. Victoria had also been seen by a practice nurse in a GP surgery of 15 years' experience who had no child protection training. In the early hours of 25 February 2000 Victoria was transferred to paediatric intensive care at St Mary's Hospital, Paddington with severe hypothermia and multiple system failure. It was to be the last of previous hospital admissions for Victoria, and one she would not return alive from. Victoria was declared dead at 3.15 p.m. on 25 February 2000. She was eight years and three months old (Laming, 2003: 3.81).

Lord Laming (2003) led the inquiry into the death of Victoria Climbié. He made 108 recommendations in total including:

- A national database of all children accessible to all professionals: 'Contact Point';
- That child protection cannot be separated from policies to improve children's lives as a whole, there is a need for services for every child and more targeted services for those with additional needs;
- A need for improved inter-agency working, communication and documentation;
- A framework to cover children and young people from birth to 19.

The inquiry and Lord Laming's recommendations led to:

- *Every Child Matters* 2003
- The Children Act 2004
- A Children's Commissioner for England.

The new Children Act 2004 included the addition of a Children's Commissioner for England. It was proposed that the Children's Commissioner would act as a voice and promote children and young people's awareness and views. There would be a concentrated focus on and response to the outcomes children and young people have said are important. The Office of the Children's Commissioner uses the United Nations Convention on the Rights of the Child (UNCRC, 1989) to guide their work.

Under the new Children Act 2004 all local authorities had to arrange, promote and cooperate between agencies; for example, health, justice, education and social services. This is the core of inter-agency working. Agencies now have a duty to ensure they have safeguarding children arrangements and that they are promoting children's welfare. All practitioners, front-line, senior and operational managers have a responsibility for safeguarding training. The *Staying Safe: Action Plan* (DCSF, 2008) included raising awareness of safeguarding and promotion of better understanding of safeguarding issues. A change should be encouraged in behaviour towards children and young people's safety and welfare. Effective coordination across government and coherent work needed to be ensured. Agencies consist of individuals who need to know how to respond effectively when faced with child protection concerns.

Comparing Maria Colwell and Victoria Climbié

It is useful to consider similarities and differences between the death of Maria Colwell in 1973 and Victoria Climbié in 2000. The death of Maria Colwell was the first of the modern-day child abuse inquiries and initiated the child care systems we know today, yet it was those very systems that were the subject of the Victoria Climbié inquiry. The impact of Maria's death established child protection, for the first time, as a social problem. Society together with organisations and professionals now had a responsibility to act, leading to the now familiar child protection systems (Parton, 2004). At the time medical diagnosis was a key feature in establishing the evidence that abuse had taken place, which has largely continued to this day. Evidenced in several of the high-profile cases and often leading to tragic impacts on the way cases continued to be handled especially in Cleveland and with Victoria, highlighted by Lord Laming (2003), medical diagnosis and opinion should not necessarily be treated at face value or considered uncritically (Parton, 2004).

The child protection systems were seen as part of the problem and also the solution. The inquiry report into the death of Maria was a relatively localised event whereas the inquiry into Victoria's death was seen as a global event and published on the internet, something which would have been unheard of and not possible in 1973 (Parton, 2004).

In terms of similarities and differences both Maria and Victoria had been in contact with various professionals and agencies, none of whom intervened appropriately, which reflected fundamental failures in respective organisations and individual incompetence. They both lived at home with their primary carers. Maria had a clear identity, a known mother, known address and school. Whereas with Victoria there were issues over her identity, she had no school or GP, and there was confusion over who held parental responsibility The practitioners on whom children should be able to rely were not noticing or listening but instead there was a tendency to focus on the needs and accounts of the parents and other adults.

The death of Victoria led to the inquiry by Lord Laming and subsequently *Every Child Matters: Change for Children* (DfES, 2003) and the Children Act 2004. Interestingly the current coalition government probably has less of a focus on *Every Child Matters*, created within the term of the previous government. The incumbent coalition government closed down the Department for Children and Families in 2010 and subsequently all previous government policy, concerning children and families, was migrated either to the National Archives or to the Department for Education.

Baby Peter Connelly

Despite government policy improvements and legislation that followed Victoria Climbié another high-profile case was that of baby Peter Connelly in 2007. Unlike Victoria, Peter was the subject of a child protection plan under the category of neglect with his older sister and also for Peter, physical abuse. Yet even that was not sufficient to protect him from the cruel actions of his mother, stepfather and step-uncle, which lead to his death in 2007. Peter had been seen on 60 different occasions by social workers, doctors and the police. Peter was found dead in his cot when he was 17 months old. Peter had been seen by a paediatrician in a clinic appointment and then he returned home to his abusers. His spine was broken at the time of examination but was undetected. Peter's childminder had voiced concerns about him yet of the many people noticing things about Peter, only the childminder was able to voice her disquiet (Jones, 2010).

His mother, Tracy Connelly, Stephen Barker, Peter's stepfather, and Jason Owen, Stephen Barker's brother, were found guilty and received custodial sentences in 2009. Peter's death led to the then Children's Minister requesting that Lord Laming conduct another report into child protection systems. Following on from his previous inquiry into the death of Victoria Climbié (2003), in 2009 Lord Laming's report was published: *The Protection of Children in England: A Progress Report* (2009). Lord Laming acknowledged there continued to be challenges; he was tasked with evaluating good practice since his previous inquiry, identifying barriers and recommending actions. His recommendations were in several areas and included: leadership and accountability, support for children, inter-agency working and the children's workforce. Included was a greater emphasis on Ofsted and monitoring how prominently schools are taking forward their safeguarding responsibilities.

Rochdale

In Rochdale in 2012 criminal proceedings were in place to prosecute a number of men accused of the sexual exploitation of young girls. At the same time the Rochdale Safeguarding Children Board (2012) produced a report which was a preliminary review of how agencies in the area worked together to safeguard children and young people at risk of sexual exploitation. It was not until 2007 that awareness of child exploitation and the scale of the problem was starting to become clear. The review found that professionals were not skilled in either recognising or responding to child sexual exploitation. Yet the report identified 50 children and young people, largely girls between 10 and 17 years old. Half were in education and half were looked after children. The general view was that while many of the children were supported by the crisis intervention team and the drug and alcohol service, the children who came into contact with social care were deemed to be 'making their own choices' and 'engaging in consensual sexual activity' and thereby not interpreted as meeting the 'thresholds' of significant harm. Despite the above teams making referrals to children's social care, referrals were not acted upon, neither was knowledge passed to the police. Nor did the teams referring to children's social care escalate their concerns when referrals were not being acted upon. It was felt that front-line practitioners and managers in children's social care did not consistently recognise or understand the nature of the sexual exploitation of young people. This was in keeping with the Barnardo's (2011) report that child sexual exploitation was not recognised as a mainstream child protection issue. The review felt that, overall, child welfare organisations missed opportunities to provide timely comprehensive responses and that the criminal justice system missed opportunities to bring the perpetrators to justice. Had they done so more children could have been protected from their criminal behaviours. It took until 2012 to finally bring the perpetrators to trial where convictions were obtained.

Edlington

What become known as the Edlington case concerned two brothers aged 10 and 11 at the time of their arrest which followed the two brothers' assault on two other young boys in Edlington, Yorkshire in 2009. They strangled, beat and forced their victims to sexually abuse each other, leaving one close to death. The brothers were subject to a child protection plan under the category of physical abuse and neglect. The Serious Case Review conducted by Doncaster Safeguarding Children Board (2010) found that local agencies had failed over years to achieve better outcomes for the brothers and therefore had failed to prevent the assaults (see also Department for Education, 2012b). In 2012 a review of the case was published: *The Edlington Case: A Review by Lord Carlile of Berriew CBE QC at the Request of The Rt Hon Michael Gove MP Secretary of State for Education* (Carlile, 2012). He highlighted there were numerous recorded related issues with the brothers going back over a period of four years when they were 6 and 7 at the time. Incidents included aggressive behaviour and assaults on other children and staff at school to name a few. Lord Carlile made a number of recommendations which have significant implications for all services involved with children and young people. Most importantly, he recommended much closer integration between services and agencies particularly health and education. Yet we are beginning to see fragmentation and moves further delineating health and education. Lord Carlile's other recommendations included keeping the responsibility for excluded children with the school implementing the exclusion. Teaching staff should undertake child development and safeguarding training. He identified that health has an essential role with regard to safeguarding and recommends increased and improved access to CAMHS, basic medicals and increased school nurse provision. Lord Carlile felt that assumptions of 'the family' being the best place for children, as enshrined in the Children Act 1989, should be challenged. The other important principle of 'best interest' should also be challenged and he felt that it is, and was not in the case of the Edlington brothers in their 'best interest' to remain for so long in the toxic family setting. Lord Carlile further recommended that greater emphasis be placed on the characteristics of the family and most significantly that children should not be accommodated as a last resort but much earlier on. His recommendations also concur with current policy of trying to ensure that babies and children who may enter the adopted system are placed with new families much earlier and the process speeded up. There is now universal recognition of the effect of trauma and abuse on the developing brain and thus child development as discussed in more detail in Chapter 2.

SAFEGUARDING CHILDREN BOARDS AND SERIOUS CASE REVIEWS

Safeguarding Children Boards are useful points of information regarding safeguarding in your locality. They have a role to promote safeguarding as a shared responsibility throughout all organisations, agencies and the wider community (Barker and Hodes, 2007).

Local Safeguarding Children Boards are responsible for conducting Serious Case Reviews (SCR). These are undertaken when a child dies, either by death or suicide and where abuse or neglect is known or suspected to be a factor, irrespective of whether children's services have been involved. They can also be convened in circumstances where a child has been seriously harmed and the case gives rise to concerns about the way in which local professionals and services worked together to safeguard and promote the welfare of children.

> From 2013 there will be a national panel of independent experts to advise LSCBs about the initiation and publication of SCRs. The role of the panel will be to support LSCBs in ensuring that appropriate action is taken to learn from serious incidents in all cases where the statutory SCR criteria are met and to ensure that those lessons are shared through publication of final SCR reports. (DfE, 2013: 69)

In the Rochdale case of sexually exploited children (Rochdale Safeguarding Children Board, 2012), the Board took the decision to undertake a preliminary review of how partner agencies responded to allegations made by the young people.

WORKING TOGETHER AND *EVERY CHILD MATTERS*

Other relevant legislation and policy includes *Working Together to Safeguard Children: A Guide to Inter-agency Working to Safeguard and Promote the Welfare of Children* (DfE, 2013). *Working Together* was first published by the Department of Health in 1999 and was continually updated, latterly in 2013. The most recent revision followed the Munro (2011) review and now includes language such as 'early help' and a 'child centred approach' as recommended by Munro's review. *Working Together* clarifies the core legal requirements, making it much clearer what individuals and organisations should do to keep children safe and promote their welfare. It is intended to provide a national framework within which agencies and professionals at local level draw up and agree on their own ways of working together to safeguard and promote the welfare of children (DfE, 2013).

Working Together defines and describes the different categories of abuse which are: physical, sexual, neglect, emotional and failure to thrive, which will be detailed later in the chapter. The *Staying Safe: Action Plan* (DCSF, 2008) followed the Children's Plan (2007). Themes from *Working Together to Safeguard Children* (2010) are based on the *Every Child Matters* (DfES, 2003) outcomes, and include: all children should achieve their potential and be physically and mentally as normal as possible. They should be able to benefit from high-quality education and live in a safe environment protected from harm. Children and young people should experience emotional wellbeing; feel loved, valued and supported by a network of reliable, affectionate relationships. They should feel competent in self-care and have a positive image and a secure sense of identity, whilst also being able to develop good interpersonal skills and confidence in social situations (Hobart and Frankel, 2005).

CHILD PROTECTION PLANS

Child protection registers became renamed in England as 'subject to child protection plans' in 2008. There are currently, as of 31 March 2012, 42,850 children subject to child protection plans under the category of abuse in England (NSPCC, 2013). It is worth remembering that sadly on average every 10 days in England and Wales, one child dies at the hand of his or her parents. Death rates for children have remained similar for the past 30 years (NSPCC, 2008). A child protection plan is not necessarily a record of child abuse but rather about a child in need of a protection plan. It should state what the intended outcomes are and what everyone is working towards. Child protection plans have core group members consisting of the parents, the child or young person, and professionals working directly with the child such as teachers or health professionals. The core group would be led by a key worker, the child's social worker. Regular meetings are held including a child protection review conference which takes place every six months. Children can remain subject to a child protection plan for over six months and over two years in some cases. It has to be remembered the potential for extreme vulnerability of children without child protection plans, of which there are many. Frequently children will not meet 'thresholds', a strategy criticised by Munro. According to the Children Act 1989 the concept of *significant harm* serves as the threshold justifying compulsory intervention. Under s.31(9) of the same Act: 'harm' means ill-treatment or the impairment of health or development; 'development' means physical, intellectual, emotional, social or behavioural development; 'health' means physical or mental health; and 'ill-treatment' includes sexual abuse and forms of ill-treatment which are not physical. Under s.31(10) of the Act: 'where the question of whether harm suffered by a child is significant turns on the child's health or development, his health or development shall be compared with that which could reasonably be expected of a similar child' (Department for Education, 2006). It has to be considered that these are open to variable interpretations, often leaving already vulnerable children in unsafe situations where they become highly vulnerable.

With regard to inter-agency working, all referrals to Children's Services must be followed up by them with an initial assessment by a social worker, which must include direct involvement with the child or young person and their family. This should then be followed up by direct engagement and feedback to the referring professional.

THE COMMON ASSESSMENT FRAMEWORK

In 2006 the Common Assessment Framework (CAF) was introduced as an assessment tool and as a standardised way of assessing a child or young person's needs. It was designed to identify early on children and young people who are vulnerable and who may benefit from additional services from health, social care or education. It must be remembered that a CAF is for a child in need, not a child at risk from harm. Neither is it a risk assessment tool. It has a focus on three areas: developmental needs, parenting capacity and family and environmental factors. It articulates with the five desired outcomes from *Every Child Matters* (DfES, 2003) and can be completed if it is thought achievement of those outcomes is hindered without additional support from universal services. It is not a referral but rather a request for further support from services. It is an ongoing assessment evolving and developing according to need. It is seen as a collaborative assessment conducted alongside and with families by a lead professional acting as a point of contact for the family and as a coordinator of inter-agency interventions (Barker and Hodes, 2007). A lead professional is able to clarify boundaries and the varying roles and responsibilities of the various agencies ensuring the child's and family's needs can be met effectively (Walker 2008). The lead professional can typically be from health, education or social care settings, for example, teachers, school nurse, health visitor, Sure Start/ children's centre professional, family support worker, or a social worker. It is important to remember that if a CAF reveals a child or young person is at risk local safeguarding procedures must be followed.

The CAF provides a nationally standardised approach with a nationally standardised expectation of what should happen throughout agencies. It should ensure children are not subject to a lot of different assessments and that information given to children and families is properly coordinated (Gardner and Cleaver, 2009). An important principle is that all assessments are child-centred requiring direct observation and communication with the child. The archived *The Common Assessment Framework: Supporting Tools* (Department for Education, 2006) is a useful document containing case examples and guidance.

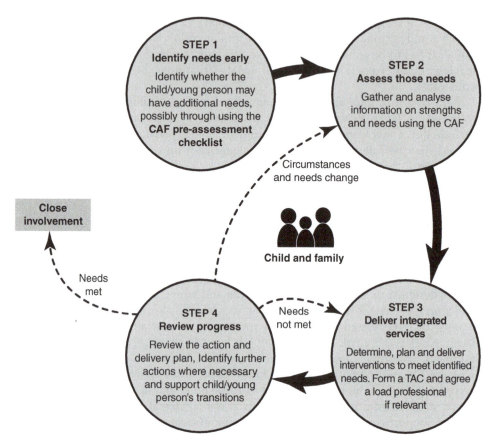

Figure 3.1   The CAF four step process

Source: Department for Education (2012a)

The Common Assessment Framework continues in use but is being strengthened by 'Family Early Help Assessment'. Early Help was introduced with the revised *Working Together to Safeguard Children* (2013). Late in 2013, 20 'Pioneering Places' were identified from the Early Intervention Foundation. In these areas CAF is being replaced by 'Early Help Assessment Framework'. Early Help retains the core themes from CAF of gathering information at a single point within an 'Early Help Hub' and using information to decide on what support is needed (Early Intervention Foundation, 2013).

CRIMINAL RECORDS BUREAU AND DISCLOSURE BARRING SERVICE CHECKS (CRB/DBS)

CRB checks were first established under Part V of the Police Act 1997 and launched in 2002. Anyone likely to have contact with children, young people and other vulnerable adults has to have CRB checks. It is estimated that 130,000 unsuitable people including rapists and paedophiles have been prevented from working with children and young people (BBC, 2013). In 2013 CRB checks were replaced by the Disclosure Barring Service (Gov. uk, 2013).

MUNRO, THE LATEST REVIEW

The most recent child protection report; The Munro Review of Child Protection: Final Report – *A child-centred system* (2011) was an independent review conducted by Professor Eileen Munro on behalf of the coalition government which came into office in 2010. The review was presented to The Secretary of State in May 2011 with 15 recommendations. These were broadly accepted by government. The three core themes are:

- Evidence has to be behind policy, namely what works which can then be implemented throughout local authorities
- Any system review must focus on the child rather than the system
- Effective protection of children and young people is about sound judgement of risk at a practice and organisational level

The review acknowledges the value of professional expertise and judgement and that 'early help' should be available where children and young people are identified as at risk. The term 'early help' is a contrast with earlier language 'early intervention' which has tended to be interpreted as early on in life. 'Early help' signifies help when problems emerge at any age (Clifton, 2013). Munro recommended that social work students need to be fully prepared for child protection work and Social Workers will now be regulated by the Health Professions Council (Blyth and Solomon, 2013). One can only wonder why this was not already an existing practice element? Why has it taken until 2011 for Munro to state what we might consider to be the obvious? What has been happening prior to her recommendation? Hopefully we can now look forward to an improved future in terms of safeguarding children and young people. Lord Laming (2009) recommended increasing numbers of Health Visitors and the coalition government set out is ambitious commitment to recruit 4,200 new Health Visitor posts by 2015. It recognises the importance and role of early intervention in improving outcomes for the future population by giving infants and children the best start possible. The plan includes preventing illness and injury and widening community support, in partnership with Sure Start centres, GP's and other health services (Department of Health, 2011). Health Visitors are in a unique position in terms of visiting and being welcomed into the homes of families with infants up to school age, with opportunity to monitor the context of the child and family. They are usually seen as non-threatening professionals supporting the health and development of mothers and infants and being able to sustain supporting relationships with families (King, 2011).

Key legislation/policy to remember

- The Children Act (1989)
- *Working Together to Safeguard Children* (2013)

- Framework for the Assessment of Children in Need and their Families (2000)
- *What to do if You are Worried a Child is Being Abused* (2006)
- *Every Child Matters* (2003)
- The Children Act (2004)
- *Staying Safe: Action Plan* (2008)

EFFECTS AND DAMAGE; WHO IS ABUSING WHOM AND WHY?

There seem to be weaknesses and bias in most research studies. It is generally considered that children in reconstituted families are overall at more risk. It is generally considered that mothers are mainly responsible for neglect and physical abuse, especially of younger children. Child sexual abusers are predominantly male with fathers or father figures being responsible for nearly all acts of interfamilial sexual abuse of children (O'Connor, 1991). Mothers are often held partly responsible in terms of being 'collusive mothers' in that they were aware of abuse taking place but did not intervene to keep children safe. In terms of interfamilial sexual abuse mothers are often passive-dependent towards the perpetrator (Meiselman, 1978, cited in O'Connor, 1991: 22). There are strong links between poverty, physical abuse and neglect. This may arise from the difficulties managing negative external factors which in turn minimises or inhibits the capacity to respond to other pressures. These external factors undoubtedly impact on maternal and infant resilience to violence (Batmanghelidjh, 2006: 94).

Abuse is considered to cross all socioeconomic groups and the links between risk factors of poverty, deprivation and abuse are strong but it must be remembered that those who are not poor, the middle and upper classes, are perhaps more efficient at hiding abuse and are less likely to be in contact with other agencies and therefore less likely to be identified. Marital discord and characteristics of the child including illness and prematurity can become sources of stress in families. Other sociological sources of stress include single-parent families who may be experiencing a lack of a support network, although interestingly all of the landmark cases considered in this chapter include children living with a mother and parental father figure and not in single-parent households. It is also worth considering that Sweden has the highest rate of single-parent households in all of the OECD countries yet scores the highest in terms of overall wellbeing in the UNICEF (2007) study.

RISK AND RESILIENCE

The risk and resilience model, as discussed in Chapter 1, acts as a reminder that in the context of safeguarding, when risk factors are chronic and severe only a minority cope. Bynner (2001) suggested that the earlier the disadvantage and the longer it has persisted the lower the likelihood of any protective factors counteracting it. We can remind ourselves that all types of abuse in childhood or adolescence constitute a risk factor in the potential development of mental health problems. However, not all abused children will develop a mental health problem. It is thought that outcomes are mitigated by subsequent supportive relationships. Given that, if abuse continues and without early intervention, risks become increased (Vostanis, 2007).

GENERATIONAL PATTERNS AND IMPACT

Ideas around intergenerational features were discussed by Kempe et al. (1985), in their paper 'The Battered Baby Syndrome'. They felt the most consistent feature in the histories of abusing families was the repetition from one generation to another. Both good and bad child-rearing patterns pass from one generation to the next in relatively unchanged form. Karr-Morse and Wiley (1997) coined the term 'ghosts from the nursery', referring to the parents who bring their own unresolved issues from their own childhoods to the rearing of their own children. Their evidence proposes that violent behaviour traits are linked to abuse and neglect in infancy. It is considered that perpetrators have certain predisposing personality and character traits. These include: low frustration tolerance, rigidity and inflexibility, aggression, punitive control, unrealistic expectations of the child and emotional immaturity, also identified by Kempe et al. (1985). So as a rule of thumb no one hurts another who has not been hurt themselves (Batmanghelidh, 2006: 155). Of course not all childhood victims of abuse go on to abuse others but most individuals in the criminal justice system as a result of violent crime and abuse of others would have almost certainly been childhood victims themselves. A recent study has demonstrated links between children exposed to family violence and changes in the brain. Changes are similar to 'combat stress' or PTSD (Post Traumatic Stress Disorder) experienced by combat soldiers. These brain changes occuring in a child's developing brain may increase vulnerability to later life stressors, increasing risks of anxiety disorders, together with a pre-disposition towards reactive aggression (McCrory et al., 2011). Indeed, it is now thought that perpetrating acts of violence against another can act as a self-soothing coping mechanism. A research study looking at early experiences of violence on brain development and the links with perpetrating violent behaviour is underway. The research is in partnership with young people as active participants, Kids Company, University College London and the Anna Freud Centre (Guinness, 2009; Anna Freud Centre, 2013). These are young people who have suffered significant harm and want to understand how and if this has impacted on any potential brain changes.

Some of the worst criminal acts have been perpetrated and carried out by children, towards other children and adults, who were abused themselves (Carlile, 2012: 47). For the individual children and young people and ultimately the adults who perpetrate abuse against others there is always a history of abuse and neglect originating in their childhood experiences. Prime examples are Tracey Connelly, Peter's mother, and the two Edlington boys who carried out acts of extreme violence against a number of other children resulting in two being left for dead. Other experiences can include frequent reconfigurations of the 'family' with departures and arrivals. Tracey Connelly grew up in a large and poor family. Her mother used alcohol no doubt as a way of numbing feeling and thinking, trying to survive extreme domestic violence from both Tracey's father and after he died Tracey's stepfather. She was unable to keep Tracey safe from increased violence from her brother. One can only consider how Tracey survived these experiences but on becoming a mother herself was not able to identify with Peter's pain or have any empathy or sympathy for him (Jones, 2010).

THE 'TOXIC TRIO'

In all of the above cases and during their own childhood there was a context and experience of domestic violence, substance misusing adults, predominantly alcohol, and often mental illness. This has been aptly described as 'toxic trio'; namely domestic violence, substance misuse and mental illness (Cleaver et al., 2009; Unwin and Hogg, 2012). The 'toxic trio' is a consistent feature of Serious Case Reviews (NSPCC, 2013). It was evident within the Serious Case Review of Daniel Pelka, although the significance of maternal mental illness did not appear to have been explored (Coventry Safeguarding Children Board 2013). Daniel grew up in an environment of domestic violence and high consumption of alcohol between his parents. His mother made two deliberate self-harm attempts which included two overdoses and walking out in front of an ambulance. She was diagnosed with clinical depression. All of these events occurred during Daniel's short lifetime and were his life experience.

It is estimated that at least 200,000 children in households reside where there is a known high risk of domestic abuse and violence (Birmingham Safeguarding Children Board, 2010). Other research carried out by YouGov 4Children puts this figure at 950,000 children affected by domestic violence, either directly as victims of violence, or indirectly in terms of witnessing violence. The impact of family violence falls heavily on women with 10% of all women experiencing domestic violence every year and two women killed each week as a result in England and Wales. It is estimated that around half of these women have children living with them (4Children, 2012).

One of the aspects looked at in UNICEF's (2007) *Child Well-being in Rich Countries* report was experiences of violence within contexts of fighting or reports of being bullied. UNICEF acknowledged this was an inadequate representation of young people's experience of violence in the countries concerned. They felt that more information on children's exposure to violence of all kinds in the home is needed. This was further highlighted as a gap, as well as the prevalence of abuse and neglect, and the well-being of looked after children, in the UNICEF (2013) report. UNICEF goes on to say that national studies show that children who often witness violence between others in the home are also most likely to be victims of violence themselves, and both forms of exposure represent incalculable levels of current misery and long-term damage to the development and wellbeing of many millions of children (UNICEF, 2003). They concluded that in some industrialised nations today as many as 1 child in every 15 is the victim of serious maltreatment and that this is an issue which needs to be dragged out from the shadows of national life and into the daylight of public and political scrutiny (UNICEF, 2007).

Neuroscience and neuropsychiatry are now providing the evidence with new findings continuing to emerge. It is now acknowledged there is a difference in the brain and the brain development of children exposed to and who have experienced abuse. In basic terms continuous bad experiences are an assault on the brain and cause disruptive functioning (Batmanghelidjh, 2007, cited in Smith, 2007). Early intervention is essential in order to minimise long-term effects, now being recognised and finally forming part of local and central government policy. Although it is interesting to note that the Munro report uses the term 'early help', which is perhaps more appropriate and does not just refer to infants but adolescents also in need of help and support.

THE 'FAMILY'

Certainly in the past 40 years since Maria Colwell's death in 1973 there has been a considerable shift in what we consider 'family' to be, reflecting social and cultural change. The 'family' is considered to be the safest and most acceptable unit in which to raise children and is globally considered to be the natural fundamental unit of society. There is a basic assumption that the family is the natural environment for the growth and wellbeing of its members, especially children. There is universal recognition that the family has the greatest potential to protect, nurture and provide. Family privacy and autonomy is valued throughout societies and the right to family life is enshrined in human rights law. But for some children 'family' can be one of the most dangerous settings to be in. Violence against children by parents and other family members has been documented globally and within the case studies considered in this chapter. As we have seen this can include physical, sexual and psychological violence as well as deliberate neglect. From infancy until 18 children are vulnerable to various forms of violence within the home, often experiencing physical, cruel or humiliating punishment in the context of discipline. Insults, name-calling, isolation, rejection, threats, emotional indifference and belittling are all forms of violence that can damage a child's emotional wellbeing. Children are most frequently sexually abused by someone they know, often a member of their own family.

BEING VIGILANT

All workers need to be vigilant in recognition of potential abuse and importantly, know how to respond. It has been noted that since the Peter Connelly case in 2007 there has been as much as a 62% increase in local authority care applications (Cafcass, 2012). It is without doubt a positive move that more concerns are being raised earlier and acted upon. However it has been highlighted that perhaps there has been a shift away from vigilance towards older children and young people as highlighted in Rochdale and other recent cases. This was consistent in the case of 'Suzie', one of the cases highlighted in the Rochdale review. Children's Social Care had not considered Suzie to be at risk of significant harm, rather it was concluded she had made a 'lifestyle' choice to be sexually active with adults. Yet as a teenager once she became pregnant, the focus from Children's Social Care was on the unborn baby for whom they did conduct a core assessment (Rochdale Safeguarding Children Board, 2012). Moving the focus to babies and away from adolescents was further borne out by the Barnardo's (2011) report into the sexual exploitation of children.

Lord Laming's (2003) inquiry into the death of Victoria Climbié highlighted gaps in the competence of staff in the statutory agencies and he stated that:

> ... effective support for children and families cannot be achieved by a single agency working alone it is a multi-disciplinary task. (Laming, 2003: 1.30)

This was further included in the *National Service Framework for Children, Young People and Maternity Services* (Department of Health and Department for Education, 2004). It was identified there were issues in identifying serious child protection issues and that there was inadequate recording and management of information systems. There needed to be a commitment that agencies and staff would work together and that:

- All staff need to be alert and able to recognise children and young people at risk of abuse;
- They are competent in recognising when a child or young person's welfare or development is impaired and/or at risk from suffering harm;
- All staff are alert to messages both verbal/non-verbal and know how to respond and communicate;
- Disabled children and young people are at higher risk of being abused.

The *National Service Framework* further set out a commitment that providers of primary care and primary care workers have a duty to promote children and young people's welfare and to prevent children from being abused or neglected and to also identify those at risk and to take appropriate action, in terms of referral to Children's Services and the police (Cleaver et al., 2009).

It is an important point that workers are not responsible for concluding or deciding whether abuse has happened but they have a responsibility to be aware of child protection procedures and know how to act appropriately if suspicious. Knowing how to respond to concerns is crucial. Very often we have instinctive responses that something is not 'quite right'. Maintaining curiosity is an important stance and something not to be ignored. It is also important to understand that disclosure will not necessarily happen. I have worked with children and young people, often for long periods of time, who present with significant mental health problems such as eating disorders, suicidal and self-harming behaviours. A few children do disclose, but often after a long period of time, years may elapse. Some young people never disclose at all. A clue is always there in terms of behaviour especially when considering children and adolescents. We need to be attentive towards any changes in behaviour beyond what would be considered developmentally 'normal' or out of character. *Working Together to Safeguard Children* (DfE, 2013a: 85–6) defines abuse under the following categories:

Abuse: A form of maltreatment of a child. Somebody may abuse or neglect a child by inflicting harm, or by failing to act to prevent harm. Children may be abused in a family or in an institutional or community setting by those known to them or, more rarely, by others (e.g. via the internet). They may be abused by an adult or adults, or another child or children.

Physical abuse: A form of abuse which may involve hitting, shaking, throwing, poisoning, burning or scalding, drowning, suffocating or otherwise causing physical harm to a child. Physical harm may also be caused when a parent or carer fabricates the symptoms of, or deliberately induces, illness in a child.

Emotional abuse: The persistent emotional maltreatment of a child such as to cause severe and persistent adverse effects on the child's emotional development. It may involve conveying to a child that they are worthless or unloved, inadequate, or valued only insofar as they meet the needs of another person. It may include not giving the child opportunities to express their views, deliberately silencing them or 'making fun' of what they say or how they communicate. It may feature age or developmentally inappropriate expectations being imposed on children. These may include interactions that are beyond the child's developmental capability, as well as overprotection and limitation of exploration and learning, or preventing the child participating in normal social interaction. It may involve seeing or hearing the ill-treatment of another. It may involve serious bullying (including cyber bullying), causing children frequently to feel frightened or in danger, or the exploitation or corruption of children. Some level of emotional abuse is involved in all types of maltreatment of a child, though it may occur alone.

Sexual abuse: Involves forcing or enticing a child or young person to take part in sexual activities, not necessarily involving a high level of violence, whether or not the child is aware of what is happening. The activities may involve physical contact, including assault by penetration (for example, rape or oral sex) or non-penetrative acts such as masturbation, kissing, rubbing and touching outside of clothing. They may also include non-contact activities, such as involving children in looking at, or in the production of, sexual images, watching sexual activities, encouraging children to behave in sexually inappropriate ways, or grooming a child in preparation for abuse (including via the internet). Sexual abuse is not solely perpetrated by adult males. Women can also commit acts of sexual abuse, as can other children.

Neglect: The persistent failure to meet a child's basic physical and/or psychological needs, likely to result in the serious impairment of the child's health or development. Neglect may occur during pregnancy as a result of maternal substance abuse. Once a child is born, neglect may involve a parent or carer failing to:

- provide adequate food, clothing, shelter (including exclusion from home or abandonment);
- protect a child from physical and emotional harm or danger;
- ensure adequate supervision (including the use of inadequate care-givers); or
- ensure access to appropriate medical care or treatment. It may also include neglect of, or unresponsiveness to, a child's basic emotional needs.

HOW TO RESPOND, KNOWING WHAT TO DO

If you suspect a baby, child or young person is being abused you have a duty and responsibility to respond. A discussion should take place with the designated individual within your organisation or your mentor (if you are a student), supervisor or line manager. The organisation concerned will have safeguarding guidance and policy. It would need to happen straightaway. If a child or young person makes a disclosure it is of paramount importance to acknowledge with the young person what has been shared. Listen and hear what is being said and acknowledge the child or young person placing their trust in you to help them. Very often children and young people disclose with the knowledge the person they are disclosing to will have a responsibility to act. Sometimes a child or young person may ask you if you can keep 'a secret'. It is vital to again hear and listen with empathy whilst telling them you will have to share the information with your supervisor (for example) and what is of paramount importance is their safety. Others you might need to speak with could be the child protection named individual within your organisation, children's social care, or the police, if there are immediate safety issues. The Nursing and Midwifery Council (2008) code of conduct is a useful point of reference with application for all workers and professionals. It states that information must be disclosed if you believe someone is at risk from harm. Consider the information regarding consent and confidentiality already discussed above. As we have seen from the cases discussed in the chapter and even when children are subject to a child protection plan they are not always safe and certainly those without a plan are highly vulnerable. The following is a guide about what to do:

- Acknowledgement
- Discuss with supervisor/manager
- Referral to Children's Services (consult local CS for procedure)
- Can telephone local Children's Duty Team for advice
- Initial child protection conference; symbolic of multi-agency working
- Decision will be made re: child protection plan
- Review within four months or earlier, then every six months. (HM Government's [2006] *What to Do if You're Worried a Child is Being Abused* and NICE (2009, modified 2013) *When to Suspect Child Maltreatment* are useful reference documents.)

It is of paramount importance to continue to support the young person. Depending on the setting it would be important to have regular face-to-face conversations and that the young person knows you are there to continue to support him or her. If Children's Services have accepted the referral they will be getting on with their assessment. It is important for you to remain in a supporting position even though you are not directly involved in any child protection proceedings. Listening and hearing the child or young person as an active participant is an important principle. You may wish to discuss other referrals, for example for counselling support, depending on the need and what is in best interest for the young person.

Sadly it is true that some children who do disclose end up being in a worse position. This was clear from the Rochdale events and the case of 'Suzie'. Despite appropriate referrals to Children's Social Care it was decided not to proceed to a child protection plan. Suzie's position remained not only as it was before referral, i.e. vulnerable, but her vulnerability would have increased in the knowledge no action was going to be taken to protect her, and particularly so if her perpetrators had that knowledge. It can be very difficult for children remaining in situations where they have alleged abuse yet despite this they may not meet thresholds whereby protective action is taken. The strategy of 'thresholds' was criticised by Munro (2011).

CHILDREN'S RIGHTS

It is important to remember children have rights as do all human beings and to briefly consider 'rights' with the context of this chapter.

> The idea of children's rights, then, may be a beacon guiding the way to the future – but it is also illuminating how many adults neglect their responsibilities towards children and how children are too often the victims of the ugliest and most shameful of human activities. (Kofi Annan, UN Secretary-General, 2001, cited in Alderson, 2008: 13)

There is often controversy and confusion about what child 'rights' actually are. Children's rights are enshrined within the *United Nations Convention on the Rights of the Child* (UNCRC, 1989). The UNCRC became the first legally binding international instrument, to incorporate the full range of human rights: civil, cultural, economic, political and social rights. It was felt that children and young people under the age of 18 needed a special convention. By 2005 nearly all states were parties except the USA and Somalia. The USA, although a signatory has not yet ratified the Convention, taking the position that the American Constitution applies to all ages with no need for a separate instrument for children. With regard to Somalia, it is not a signatory because of the practice of female genital mutilation.

It is also worth noting that historically children and young people were not considered independent until the 19th century but rather the 'property' of another. The Married Women's Property Act in the late 19th century gave separate rights to women for the first time, prior to which women were considered the property of another. Think about other similarities for women and children in other cultures and countries and the implications when specific cultures disperse globally through migration, to the UK for instance. Children's rights can be seriously compromised in relation to issues of forced marriages, female and male circumcision and Ashura in the Shi'a Muslim community (which involves flagellation). Harmful traditional practices are generally imposed on children at an early age by family or community leaders (United Nations Secretary General's Study, 2006). There have been recent cases in England highlighted in the media of male circumcision carried out on infants in the community with fateful outcomes. Much of this violence is hidden behind closed doors or because of shame or fear. Sadly, experiences and exposure to violence is more prevalent in the family than outside the family.

Activity

Do you think infant male circumcision is a safeguarding and/or children's rights issue?

Infant male circumcision takes place for religious rather than medical reasons so can be considered a ritual rather than a therapeutic procedure. It continues throughout the world despite other rituals like female circumcision and facial scarification being made illegal (Hinchley, 2007). The debate revolves around parental beliefs versus the rights of the child. Controversy surrounds human rights and the Human Rights Act 1998, which upholds freedoms to practise religious and cultural beliefs and uphold family life (Articles 8 and 9), and the UNCRC (1989: Articles 19 and 24). Article 19 is about protection from injury and abuse, Article 24 relates to the abolition of traditional practices prejudicial to children's health. Clearly infants do not have the capacity to consent so should the procedure be carried out regardless? It is not a risk free procedure as recently highlighted by the death of an infant (Boyle et al., 2000; Kasprzak, 2012).

The UNCRC continues to underpin policy and practice throughout many organisations and governments today. The Convention was cited in recent child abuse reports and inquiries. There are 54 articles and all signatories agree to develop and undertake all actions and policies in the light of *best interest* of the child. For example, and in relation to this chapter, Article 2 states children and young people should be *protected from all forms of punishment* and Article 19, from all *forms of physical or mental violence*. Article 12 is about the right to *express views freely in all matters*. The UNCRC reflects a new vision with children no longer being the property of adults and offers a vision of the child as an individual and as a member of a family and a community with age-appropriate rights and responsibilities. There is now a focus on the whole child with a demand for a basic quality of life for all children not just a privileged few. However, this is only a reality when respected throughout families, institutions, education, communities and all who provide services for children. The role of implementation of the UNCRC was granted to UNICEF with a legal obligation to promote and protect child rights.

The UNCRC and *Every Child Matters*

It is interesting to consider both *Every Child Matters* (DfES, 2003) and the UNCRC (1989) in terms of what they give children. The UNCRC (1989) sets out 40 substantive rights on all aspects of childhood with a clear set of entitlements and comprehensive legal obligations. These are based on broad principles with potential different applications in different cultures (Alderson, 2008). *Every Child Matters* (DfES, 2003), on the other hand, has five outcome goals which are open to wide interpretation and discretion with no legal obligations. UNICEF mapped the UNCRC articles against the five *Every Child Matters* outcomes (UNCRC, 2006). There are three themes underpinning all the UNCRC articles (1989): rights to health (*provision*), rights to protection from safety and harm (*protection*) and the right to be heard (*participation*). If you consider the high-profile cases discussed in this chapter it is not difficult to see that even basic human rights were not afforded to those children.

Participation and the child's voice (UNCRC Article 12)

Eileen Munro's (2011) review acknowledged that often the voice of the child is overlooked and this must now change. That was certainly apparent in the other high-profile inquiries. Victoria Climbié was never spoken to in her own language. The children in the Cleveland inquiry had decisions made for them by medical staff. The voices of 250 children were included and acknowledged in Munro's review, which is a refreshing emphasis in terms of children's rights. Whilst the UNCRC articles are internationally recognised and were ratified in the UK in 1991 their influence and reach is at times limited. Article 12 is about the child's voice and views being respected, modelled in the Munro review process itself. It is encouraging that the coalition government recognises the importance of the UNCRC as underpinning our child protection system (Department for Education, 2011).

Activity

What ideas do you have around smacking children? Should children be protected in law? Should parents be criminalised if they physically chastise their children? What about 'best interest' and is there a conflict?

'Best interest' has different applications in different societies and cultures. It is an important guiding principle of the Children Act 1989 and for organisations, agencies and workers to be acting in 'best interest' at all times. There is a continuing debate over physical chastisement of children. In many countries, particularly in Europe, smacking children is against the law yet the UK, Australia, Canada and the USA maintain it is lawful. There continues to be ideas of 'ownership' to this day and that parents should make their own decisions about discipline regarding their children. Not all deem it the role of the state to intervene. Indeed the Children Act 2004 uses terminology such as 'reasonable chastisement' and advises that a mark should not be left if a parent chooses to smack their child. Children are the only group of people not to be protected by law in the UK. If one smacked an adult one would rightly be liable to arrest and be subject to a charge of common assault. However, smacking one's own children would not lead to such an outcome beyond the legal framework of the Children Act 2004, as above. The picture is rather conflicting and confusing given the *Every Child Matters* (DfES, 2003) policy and one of the goals being 'staying safe', and that since in 1991 the UK government ratified the UNCRC (1989). So there would appear to be a misfit and inconsistency with UK legislation and government policy. It is also interesting to note that the UK has outlawed corporal punishment in schools yet not behind the closed doors of 'the home', which includes the homes of children with foster parents.

CONSENT

It is important to consider both consent and confidentiality and to be able to apply some clarity and understanding, not only when considering child protection and safeguarding, but when working generally with children, young people and families. Consent and confidentiality frequently become an issue in health care settings but not exclusively. The principle of consent is a cornerstone of medical ethics and is enshrined in international human rights law and the UNCRC (1989) as discussed above. Consent must be informed, which means the person giving consent understands why the information needs to be shared. In health settings consent is about expressing permission before any medical treatment can be carried out. Children and young people are on a continuum from an incompetent minor to a legally competent adult. With babies and children consent is usually obtained from someone with parental responsibility. It is important to understand what is known as 'Gillick competency'. Victoria Gillick sought assurances that contraceptives would never be prescribed for her children below 16 without her consent. The case went to the High Court (*Gillick* v *West Norfolk and Wisbech Area Health Authority* 1982) and eventually the House of Lords, where Lord Scarman finally ruled in 1985 that:

... whether or not a child is capable of giving the necessary consent will depend on the child's maturity and understanding and the nature of the consent required. The child must be capable of making a reasonable assessment of the advantages and disadvantages of the treatment proposed, so the consent, if given, can be properly and fairly described as true consent.

This was an important ruling which continues in use today. At the same time Lord Fraser set out guidance, known as the 'Fraser guidelines' aimed at professionals and at the time of the ruling, primarily concerning contraception. They are now considered to have application to a range of interventions, but with acknowledgement that the level of maturity/understanding needed increases with the complexity of the intervention. The guiding principle should be the professionals' own code and what is in *best interest* for the child or young person.

Activity

Elizabeth is 13. She is refusing life-saving treatment of a heart transplant. Elizabeth has spent most of her life in and out of hospital with a chronic heart condition. Elizabeth is an intelligent young person who despite her numerous hospitalisations and interventions has kept up with her school work, hobbies and friends. Her parents have consented but Elizabeth is refusing a heart transplant.

Can Elizabeth's health care team proceed without her consent but with her parents' consent?

They would not be able to proceed if Elizabeth refuses to consent. She would be covered by 'Gillick competency' rules as above. Parental consent alone would not be enough if Elizabeth is refusing treatment. The health care Trust concerned might apply to the court for a ward of court and a judge would make a decision. In a similar case in 2008 an application to the court by a Trust was turned down (see BBC, 2008). The young person involved, Hannah, changed her mind and underwent the recommend procedure and has survived (BBC, 2010). Hannah and her mother went on to write a book called *Hannah's Choice* (Jones and Jones, 2010).

CONFIDENTIALITY

A duty of confidence arises when one person discloses information to another in circumstances where it is reasonable to expect that the information will be held in confidence. It is a legal obligation that is derived from case law; it is a requirement established within professional codes of conduct throughout all professions. With regard to the NHS, patient information is generally held under legal and ethical obligations of confidentiality. Information provided in confidence should not be used or disclosed in a form that might identify a patient without his or her consent

(Department of Health, 2003). Children and young people as well as adults are enti-tled to the same duties of confidence covered by common laws of confidentiality, the Data Protection Act 1998, the Human Rights Act 1998 and administrative law. Information sharing is subject to current debate and there is often confusion when records and information held by one agency cannot be shared by another. With regard to child protection, issues of safeguarding override confidentiality and would be the only time confidentiality would be breached if consent could not be obtained. Caldicott (1997) principles govern information sharing particularly in health settings but also extended to social care settings. The underlying principle is that the sharing of information between professionals is essential to enable early help for children and to safeguard and promote the welfare of children (Walker, 2008). Information sharing is potentially a greater emerging problem and may put children at increased risk, especially with continued decentralisation of agencies to local levels and the 'silo mentality' of health education and social care. This has recently been illustrated by the recent government proposal for a NHS database of children attending accident and emergency departments. Lord Laming's recommendation of a national database 'Contact Point', shared across all agencies, as he suggested in 2003, has not become a reality, nor is it likely to be, given the rights and civil liberties agenda.

Activity

Sasha is 15 and in A&E following an episode of self-harm. She has consented to the treatment of her physical wounds. As per NICE (2004) guidelines and local policy she has been admitted to the paediatric ward at the hospital to await assessment by Tier 3 CAMHS. This the fourth time in the last two months she has been seen in A&E for self-harm, last time she took an overdose of paracetamol. Sasha does not want her parents to know.

Do her parents need to be notified? Explain your response.

According to Gillick, Sasha is competent and does understand what has happened to her. However it would not be good practice to go along with Sasha's request to not tell her parents and Caldicott principles would apply 'justify the purpose' and 'best interest' from the Children Act and UNCRC 1989. There may possibly be a case for not doing so had it been a first admission but this is the fourth occasion for Sasha and given what we know from research Sasha is at a high risk of a completed suicide. Therefore informing parents could be justified on the grounds of a risk of significant harm and a threat to her life. Breaching confidentiality would be on the same grounds. The decision would be made however in consultation both with Sasha the A&E team and the CAMHS clinician conducting the psychosocial assessment. It would not be good practice to see Sasha in isolation of her family, best practice would include thinking and working with both Sasha and her family. Understanding Sasha and her predicament in the context of her family is the best way to support her and what treatment intervention may be required.

CONCLUSION

We have certainly come some way in the last 50 years in the recognition of unacceptable behaviours towards children and there has been significant policy and legislation to protect children, yet there is still a long way to go if zero child abuse is to be achieved. We must remember the unique status of children and young people in terms of their vulnerability and our own responsibility to always act appropriately with regard to safeguarding and protecting them. All child protection cases by their very nature are complex and unique to their situation. There is no single overarching intervention for all but rather it is about interpreting and working together having timely responses that are in the best interests of children and safeguarding principles. It is also important to recognise our own duties and boundaries and when to seek help and supervision. Children will continue to be abused and sadly we will not have seen the end of inquiries. The child protection system continues to evolve in response to the inquiries and reviews and is an ever-changing landscape. It is our duty to children and young people to promote their rights, remain vigilant, make referrals, seek advice and ask questions of Children's Social Care and the Local Safeguarding Children Boards if our curiosity is not satisfied. Above all listen to children, either through conversations or by interpreting behaviours and what you see. Make it your responsibility and act accordingly please. As Lord Laming said: 'NOW JUST DO IT'.

REFERENCES

Alderson, P. (2008) *Young Children's Rights: Exploring Beliefs, Principles and Practice.* London: Jessica Kingsley.

Anna Freud Centre (2013) *The Brain Study (TBS) An Investigation of the Neural and Physiological Changes Associated with Behavioural Improvements in Young People who Receive Services from Kids Company.* Available from: www.annafreud.org/pages/the-brain-study-tbs.html (accessed January 2014).

Barker, J. and Hodes, D. (2007) *The Child in Mind A Child Protection Handbook*, 3rd edn. London: Routledge.

Barnardo's (2011) *Puppet on a String: The Urgent Need to Cut Children Free from Sexual Exploitation.* Available from: www.barnardos.org.uk/ctf_puppetonastring_report_final.pdf (accessed February 2013).

Batmanghelidjh, C. (2006) *Shattered Lives: Children who Live with Courage and Dignity.* London: Jessica Kingsley.

BBC (2008) Girl Wins Right to Refuse Heart. Available from: news.bbc.co.uk/1/hi/england/hereford/worcs/7721231.stm (accessed February 2013).

BBC (2010) Heart Refusal Girl Back at School. Available from: news.bbc.co.uk/1/hi/england/hereford/worcs/8440818.stm (accessed February 2013).

BBC (2013) Judges Rule CRB Checks 'Incompatible' with Human Rights Act. Available from: www.bbc.co.uk/news/uk-21205198 (accessed April 2013).

Birmingham Safeguarding Children Board (2010) *Serious Case Review Under Chapter VIII 'Working Together to Safeguard Children' in Respect of the Death of a Child.* Case

Number 14. Available from: www.lscbbirmingham.org.uk/downloads/Case+14.pdf (accessed January 2013).

Blyth, M. and Solomon, E. (eds) (2013) *Effective Safeguarding for Children and Young People: What Next after Munro?* Bristol: The Policy Press.

Boyle, G., Svoboda, J., Price, C. and Turner, N. (2000) Circumcision of Healthy Boys: Criminal Assault? *Journal of Law and Medicine*, 7: 301–10. Available at: www.cirp.org/library/legal/boyle1/ (accessed November 2013).

British Medical Journal (1988) Summary of the Cleveland Inquiry. 297(6642): 190–191, 16 July. Available from: www.ncbi.nlm.nih.gov/pmc/articles/PMC1834212/pdf/bmj00295-0046.pdf (accessed November 2013).

Bynner, J. (2001) Childhood Risks and Protective Factors in Social Exclusion. *Children and Society*, 15 (5): 285–301.

Cafcass (2012) *Three Weeks in November... Three Years on... Cafcass Care Application Study 2012.* Available from: www.cafcass.gov.uk/media/6437/Cafcass%20Care%20Application%20Study%202012%20FINAL.pdf (accessed August 2013).

Caldicott, F. (1997) *Report on the Review of Patient-identifiable Information.* Available from: webarchive.nationalarchives.gov.uk/+/www.dh.gov.uk/en/Publicationsandstatistics/Publications/PublicationsPolicyAndGuidance/DH_4068403 (accessed February 2013).

Carlile, Lord, (2002) 'Too Serious a Thing': a review of safeguards for Children and Young People treated and cared for by the NHS in Wales. Available from: www.wales.nhs.uk/publications/english_text.pdf (accessed November 2013). See also: http://wales.gov.uk/topics/childrenyoungpeople/rights/advocacy/model/why/?lang=en (accessed November 2013).

Carlile, Lord (2012) *The Edlington Case: A Review by Lord Carlile of Berriew CBE QC at the Request of The Rt Hon Michael Gove MP Secretary of State for Education.* Available from: www.gov.uk/government/uploads/system/uploads/attachment_data/file/177098/The_Edlington_case.pdf (accessed August 2013).

Children's Plan (2007) http://webarchive.nationalarchives.gov.uk/20130401151715/https://www.education.gov.uk/publications/eOrderingDownload/Childrens_Plan_Summary.pdf (accessed November 2013).

Cleaver, H., Cawson, P., Gorin, S. and Walker, S. (eds) (2009) *Safeguarding Children: A Shared Responsibility.* Chichester: Wiley-Blackwell.

Clifton, J. (2013) The Child's Voice in the Child Protection System. In Blyth, M. and Solomon, E. (eds) *Effective Safeguarding for Children and Young People: What Next after Munro?* Bristol: The Policy Press, pp. 51–68.

Coventry Safeguarding Children Board (2013) *Serious Case Review re Daniel Pelka, Overview Report*, available from: www.coventrylscb.org.uk/files/SCR/FINAL%20Overview%20Report%20%20DP%20130913%20Publication%20version.pdf (accessed October 2013).

Department for Children, Schools and Families (2008) *Staying Safe: Action Plan.* Available from: http://webarchive.nationalarchives.gov.uk/20130401151715/https://www.education.gov.uk/publications/eOrderingDownload/DCSF-00151-2008.pdf (accessed November 2013).

Department for Education (2006) *The Common Assessment Framework: Supporting Tools* (archived document). Available from: www.education.gov.uk/publications/standard/publicationDetail/Page1/CAF-SUPPORT-TOOLS (accessed January 2013).

Department for Education (2011) *A Child Centred System: The Government's Response to the Munro Review of Child Protection.* London: TSO. Available from: www.education.gov.uk/publications/standard/publicationDetail/Page1/DFE-00064-2011 (accessed January 2013).

Department for Education (2012a) *The Common Assessment Framework Process.* Available from: www.education.gov.uk/childrenandyoungpeople/strategy/integratedworking/caf/a0068957/the-caf-process (accessed February 2013).

Department for Education (2012b) *Serious Case Review Report: 'J' Children in Edlington.* Available from: www.education.gov.uk/a00205927/serious-case-review-report-j-children-in-edlington (accessed January 2013).

Department for Education (2013) *Working Together to Safeguard Children: A Guide to Inter-agency Working to Safeguard and Promote the Welfare of Children.* Available from: http://media.education.gov.uk/assets/files/pdf/w/working%20together.pdf (accessed October 2013).

Department of Health (2003) *Confidentiality: NHS Code of Practice.* Available from: www.dh.gov.uk/en/Publicationsandstatistics/Publications/PublicationsPolicyAndGuidance/DH_4069253 (accessed February 2013).

Department of Health and Department for Education (2004) *National Service Framework for Children, Young People and Maternity Services.* London: DH and DfE.

Department of Health (2011) *Health Visitor Implementation Plan 2011–2015: A Call to Action.* Available from: www.wp.dh.gov.uk/publications/files/2012/11/Health-visitor-implementation-plan.pdf (accessed January 2013).

DfES (Department for Education and Skills) (2003) *Every Child Matters.* London: DfES.

Doncaster Safeguarding Children Board (2010) *A Serious Case Review: The 'J' Children Executive Summary.* Available from: www.doncastersafeguardingchildren.co.uk/Images/execsumchildren_J_tcm36-68398.pdf (accessed January 2013).

Early Intervention Foundation (2013) *EIF's 'Poineering Places' Announced.* Available from: www.earlyinterventionfoundation.org.uk/media-centre/press-releases/46-eif-s-pioneering-places-announced (accessed January 2014).

4Children (2012) *The Enemy Within: 4 Million Reasons to Tackle Family Conflict and Family Violence.* Available from: www.4children.org.uk/Resources/Detail/The-Enemy-Within-Report (accessed January 2013).

Gardner, R. and Cleaver, H. (2009) Working Effectively with Parents. In Cleaver, H., Cawson, P., Gorin, S. and Walker, S. (eds) *Safeguarding Children: A Shared Responsibility.* Chichester: Wiley-Blackwell, pp. 38–61.

Gillick v Norfolk and West Wisbech Health Authority (1982) House of Lords (1985) Available from: www.bailii.org/uk/cases/UKHL/1985/7.html (accessed January 2013).

Gov.uk (2013) *Disclosure and Barring Service Checks* [previously CRB checks]. Available from: www.gov.uk/disclosure-barring-service-check (accessed April 2013).

Guinness, L. (2009) *Neuroscience Research with the Anna Freud Centre and University College London.* Available from: www.kidsco.org.uk/news-events/2009/neuroscience-research-with-the-anna-freud-centre-university-college-london (accessed February 2013).

Hendry, J. and Macinnes, M. (2011) Child Abuse and Child Protection. In Claveirole, A. and Gaughan, M. (eds) *Understanding Children and Young People's Mental Health.* Chichester: Wiley-Blackwell, pp. 132–48.

Hinchley, G. (2007) Is Infant Male Circumcision an Abuse of the Rights of the Child? Yes. *British Medical Journal,* 335 (7631): 1180.

HM Government (2006) *What to Do if You Are Worried a Child is Being Abused.* Available from: www.education.gov.uk/publications/standard/publicationdetail/page1/dfes-04320-2006 (accessed February 2013).

Hobart, C. and Frankel, J. (2005) *Good Practice in Child Protection,* 2nd edn. Cheltenham: Nelson Thornes.

Jones, A. (2010) *Working with Complex Child Protection Cases,* Paper 2, (unpublished AIMH conference paper).

Jones, H. and Jones, K. (2010) *Hannah's Choice: A Daughters Love for Life: The Mother who Let Her Make the Hardest Decision of All.* London: Harper Collins.

Karr-Morse, R. and Wiley, M. (1997) *Ghosts from the Nursery: Tracing the Roots of Violence*. New York: Atlantic Monthly Press.

Kasprzak, E. (2012) Make Home Circumcision Illegal. BBC News, 14 December. Available from: www.bbc.co.uk/news/uk-england-20527625 (accessed February 2013).

Kempe, H., Silverman, F., Steele, B., Droegemueller, W. and Silver, H. (1985) The Battered Child Syndrome. *Child Abuse and Neglect*, 9: 143–54.

King, N. (2011) *Education Committee: Children First: The Child Protection System in England (Parliamentary session)*. Available from: www.publications.parliament.uk/pa/cm201213/cmselect/cmeduc/137/137vw03.htm (accessed January 2013).

Knowles, G. (2009) *Ensuring Every Child Matters*. London: Sage.

Laming, Lord (2003) *The Victoria Climbié Inquiry: Report of an Inquiry by Lord Laming*. London: TSO. Available from: www.officialdocuments.gov.uk/document/cm57/5730/5730.pdf (accessed August 2013).

Laming, Lord (2009) *The Protection of Children in England: A Progress Report*. London: TSO. Available from: www.education.gov.uk/publications/eOrderingDownload/HC-330.pdf (accessed August 2013).

McCrory, E. J., De Brito, S. A., Sebastian, C.L., Mechelli, A., Bird, G., Kelly, P.A. and Viding, E. (2011) Heightened neural reactivity to threat in child victims of family violence. *Current Biology*, 21(23): R947–R948.

Molly, M. (2012) *Don't Ignore the Hunger on our Doorstep*. The Trussell Trust Food Bank Network. Available from: www.trusselltrust.org/resources/documents/Press/Dont-ignore-the-hunger-on-our-doorstep-warns-foodbank-charity.pdf (accessed February 2013).

Munro, E. (2011) *The Munro Review of Child Protection: Final Report – A Child Centred System*. London: TSO. Available from: www.education.gov.uk/publications/standard/publicationDetail/Page1/CM%208062 (accessed January 2013).

National Archives (2013) *7. Emigration of Children*. Available from: www.nationalarchives.gov.uk/records/research-guides/emigration.htm (accessed January 2013).

National Institute for Clinical Excellence (2004) *Self-harm: The Short-term Physical and Psychological Management and Secondary Prevention of Self-harm in Primary and Secondary Care*. Available from: www.nice.org.uk/nicemedia/pdf/CG016NICEguideline.pdf (accessed February 2013).

NICE (2009) (National Institute for Clinical Excellence) *When to Suspect Child Maltreatment*, (modified March 2013). Available from: www.nice.org.uk/nicemedia/live/12183/44914/44914.pdf (accessed October 2013).

NSPCC (2008) *NSPCC Policy Summary Child Death Investigation and Review*. Available from: www.nspcc.org.uk/Inform/policyandpublicaffairs/policysummaries/ChildDeathInvestigation_wdf57475.pdf (accessed January 2013).

NSPCC (2012) *ChildLine over 25 Years*. Available from: www.nspcc.org.uk/what-we-do/childline-25/childline-over-25-years_wda85064.html (accessed January 2013).

NSPCC (2013) *Children Subject to Child Protection Plans - England 2008–2012*. Available from: www.nspcc.org.uk/Inform/research/statistics/england_wdf49858.pdf (accessed January 2013).

Nursing and Midwifery Council (2008) *NMC Code of Conduct*. London: NMC.

O'Connor, R. (1991) *Child Sexual Abuse: Treatment, Prevention and Detection*, The Centre for Health Programme Evaluation (CHPE) Working Paper 16. Available from: www.buseco.monash.edu.au/centres/che/pubs/wp16.pdf (accessed February 2013).

Office for National Statistics (2011) *Infant and Perinatal Mortality in England and Wales 2011, Infant Deaths and Infant Mortality Rates 2000–2011 England and Wales*. Available from: www.ons.gov.uk/ons/taxonomy/index.html?nscl=Infant+Mortality (accessed January 2013).

Parton, N. (2004) From Maria Colwell to Victoria Climbié: Reflections on a Generation of Public Inquiries into Child Abuse. *Child Abuse Review*, 13 (2): 80–94. Available from: www.gptsw.net/papers/clwlclmbi.pdf (accessed January 2013).

Parton, N. (2006) *Safeguarding Childhood: Early Intervention and Surveillance in a Late Modern Society*. Basingstoke: Palgrave Macmillan.

Radford, L., Corral, S., Beadley, C., Fisher, H., Howat, N. and Collishaw, S. (2011) *Child Abuse and Neglect in the UK Today*. London: NSPCC. Available from: www.nspcc.org.uk/Inform/research/findings/child_abuse_neglect_research_PDF_wdf84181.pdf (accessed January 2013).

Rochdale Safeguarding Children Board (2012) *Review of Multi-agency Responses to the Sexual Exploitation of Children*. Available from: www.rbscb.org/CSEReport.pdf (accessed January 2013).

Skuse, D.H, (1985) Non-organic Failure to Thrive: A Reappraisal. *Archives of Disease in Childhood*, 60 (2): 173–8. Available from: http://adc.bmj.com/content/60/2/173.full.pdf (accessed April 2013).

Smith, R. (2007) Brains and Misbehaviour. *Children and Young People Now*, 31 October–6 November, pp. 20–1.

UNCRC (1989) *United Nations Convention on the Rights of the Child*. Office of the United Nations High Commissioner for Human Rights. Available from: www2.ohchr.org/english/law/crc.htm (accessed February 2013).

UNCRC (2006) *Every Child Matters: The Five Outcomes and the UN Convention on the Rights of the Child (UNCRC)*. Available from: www.education.gov.uk/publications/standard/_arc_Childrenandfamilies/Page7/32016 (accessed February 2013).

UNICEF (2003) *Report Card 5: A League Table of Child Maltreatment Deaths in Rich Countries*. Available from: www.unicef-irc.org/publications/pdf/repcard5e.pdf (accessed February 2013).

UNICEF (2007) *Report Card 7: An Overview of Child Well-being in Rich Countries*. Available from: www.unicef-irc.org/publications/pdf/rc7_eng.pdf (accessed January 2013).

UNICEF (2013) *Report Card 11: Child Well-being in Rich Countries, A Comparative Overview*. Available from: www.unicef.org.uk/Images/Compaigns/FINAL_RC11-ENG-LORS-fn12.pdf (accessed 24 February 2014).

United Nations Secretary General's Study (2006) *Violence Against Children*. Available from: www.unviolencestudy.org/ (accessed January 2013).

Unwin, P. and Hogg, R. (2012) *Effective Social Work with Children and Families: A Skills Handbook*. London: Sage.

Vostanis, P. (2007) Mental Health and Mental Disorders. In Coleman, J. and Hagell, A. (eds) *Adolescence, Risk and Resilience: Against the Odds*. Chichester: Wiley-Blackwell, pp. 89–107.

Walker, G. (2008) *Working Together for Children: A Critical Introduction to Multi-agency Working*. London: Continuum.

4

MENTAL HEALTH PROMOTION STRATEGIES WITH CHILDREN, YOUNG PEOPLE AND FAMILIES

ERICA PAVORD

Overview

- What is mental health and why do we need to promote it?
- National policy and how it promotes mental health
- National strategies which aim to promote emotional wellbeing and mental health including:
  - Midwifery and health visiting
  - The Family Nurse Partnership Programme
  - The Solihull Approach
  - Parenting programmes
  - Early Years education
  - SEAL
  - Nurture groups
  - The United Kingdom Resilience Programme
  - Anti-bullying strategies
  - Drug and alcohol education

This chapter will introduce the main mental health promotion strategies that support children, young people and families. It will explore the concept of mental health promotion, enhancing capacity for mental health and preventing mental health problems. It includes working with children, young people, parents, families, schools and communities. The potential of education to impact on mental health awareness and promotion is particularly important with its emphasis on emotional literacy and wellbeing.

In Chapter 2 you will have learned about the various stages of development and what a child needs to develop into a mentally healthy person. Chapter 6 focuses on specific interventions aimed at supporting children and adolescents who are experiencing mental health problems. This chapter will focus on the interventions made by universal services such as education services, health services and children's centres. The CAMHS Review (2008) outlined the areas which need to be focused on to improve universal and specialist services. It recommended that:

> Everybody will recognise the part they can play in helping children grow up, have a good understanding of what mental health and psychological wellbeing is and how they can promote resilience in children and young people, and know where to go if they need more information and help. (CAMH Review, 2008: 11)

It went on to recommend that

> ... universal services will play a pivotal role in promotion, prevention and early intervention.

This chapter will focus on how to encourage healthy development through mental health promotion strategies. *Healthy Lives, Healthy People* (Department of Health, 2011b), is the first public health strategy that puts mental health on an equal par with physical health and the paper entitled *No Health Without Mental Health* sets out the government's intention to improve the mental health of the population. This document describes mental wellbeing as:

> ... the ability to cope with life's problems and make the most of life's opportunities. It is about feeling good and functioning well, both as individuals and collectively. (Department of Health, 2011a: 9)

Inevitably childhood may not run smoothly and most of us at different times in our development encounter obstacles, difficulties and challenges which can affect healthy emotional development and a strong sense of identity. People's ability to cope with challenges and difficulties depends on how resilient they are and their resilience will depend on a combination of various factors such as their early childhood experiences, their environment, their education, their physical health. Chapter 1 discussed the relationship between risk and resilience and showed how individuals' ability to cope with risk factors depends on the protective factors around them. Strategies that promote mental health in children and young people are those that aim to reduce the risk factors and increase the protective factors.

WHY IS MENTAL HEALTH PROMOTION SO IMPORTANT?

Chapter 1 has shown the prevalence of mental health problems amongst children and young people but it is important to note that they are only the ones who have been seen by health services or have reported a problem. The numbers are likely to be much higher. Furthermore, the importance of focusing on children and their emotional wellbeing is highlighted when we take into account that half of adults with mental illnesses had received a diagnosis before the age of 15 (Kim-Cohen et al., 2003). The financial impact of mental illness is huge. In 2003 the Sainsbury Centre for Mental Health estimated that the economic and social costs of mental health problems in England amounted to £77.4 billion. This figure was updated to £105.2 billion in the financial year 2009/10 (Centre for Mental Health, 2010).

These statistics alone show how vitally important it is to provide services and support for children and young people and to focus on the promotion of mental health and emotional wellbeing from birth into adulthood.

Mental health promotion strategies give children, young people and their families the opportunity to strengthen wellbeing and to increase their ability to stay mentally healthy and cope with the difficulties that they face. Everyone in a community has a role to play in ensuring that the environment in which children are growing up promotes their mental health. Children, young people and families should have access to supportive environments to ensure that mental health is promoted. Schools and health services are in the ideal position to promote mental health and to recognise children's emerging needs. Recognising the needs and providing specific support to vulnerable children, young people and families is particularly important as they are more at risk of developing mental health problems than the general population. It might be more accurate to call these strategies 'prevention' rather than 'promotion' and it is useful to understand this distinction. Mental health *promotion* strategies are wide reaching and might not specifically target those groups that are most at risk of developing mental illnesses. Strategies aimed at *prevention* of mental illness will target particular groups that are more vulnerable and are exposed to a greater number of risk factors. An example of this might be the delivery of Personal, Social and Health Education (PSHE) lessons in schools that address the emotional wellbeing of all pupils; this is a universal strategy that reaches all children and young people in schools. A more targeted approach would be a nurture group in a school which aims to improve the confidence and resilience of vulnerable pupils (Nurture Groups, n.d.). Dwivedi and Brinley Harper (2004) argue that it is less relevant to distinguish between promotion and prevention when it comes to children as programmes that focus on the healthy emotional development of children can have important preventative effects.

TACKLING STIGMA

One of the greatest challenges facing strategies and projects that aim to prevent mental ill health is the attitude that society still has towards mental illness. By the time a child is halfway through primary school he or she may have a rich and usually derogatory vocabulary to describe people with a mental illness. The media often represent people with mental health problems as dangerous and frightening or ridiculous, weak and ineffectual. The stigma attached to mental illness means that those who are experiencing or at risk of developing a mental illness are less likely to seek help for fear of ridicule and rejection. One of the aims of promoting mental health should be to explore and challenge people's attitudes towards mental ill health and the stereotypes and misconceptions that surround it.

The charities Mind and Rethink Mental Illness run the leading stigma and anti-discrimination campaign to challenge attitudes to mental illness. The Time to Change campaign, funded by the government and Comic Relief, runs events and campaigns encouraging the public to change their attitudes and behaviour towards people with mental health problems (Time to Change, 2012).

Activity

The media can be a powerful tool in either creating or tackling stigma around mental illness. What have you seen in the media – news or drama – which has highlighted some of the issues around mental illness? Would you say that this has helped or hindered the campaign to tackle the stigma of mental illness?

MENTAL HEALTH PROMOTION POLICY

Mental health promotion strategies have to target the population at three levels:

Structural/policy: developing initiatives to reduce discrimination and inequalities, to promote access to education, meaningful employment, affordable housing, health, social and other services which support those who are vulnerable. Examples of this might be the Pupil Premium that aims to address the inequalities in schools between children from poorer backgrounds and their wealthier peers by allocating extra funding to children who receive free school meals.

Community: increasing social support, social inclusion and participation, improving neighbourhood environments, anti-bullying strategies at school, workplace health, community safety, child care and self-help networks. Examples of this might be children's centres offering child care and groups that promote health and wellbeing.

Individual: this would include strategies which aim to increase emotional resilience through interventions designed to promote self-esteem, life and coping skills, e.g. communicating, negotiating, relationship and parenting skills. Examples of this might be school clubs that promote positive friendships, problem solving and self-esteem.

This chapter will focus mainly on Tier 1 services that promote mental health to individuals and within communities such as health visitors, midwives, Early Years providers, schools, youth work, police, GPs. It is not possible to cover even a fraction of the different strategies, projects and programmes that exist nationwide and aim to promote mental health for children and young people so this chapter will look at a just a few of the strategies that are targeted at the general population.

Before looking at specific strategies and programmes, it is important to have a knowledge and understanding of the policy that underpins the provision and delivery of mental health promotion strategies. The policy outlined is based on England and it should be remembered that the devolved governments of Wales, Scotland and Northern Ireland will have their own policy documents.

An overview of policy

2003

Every Child Matters: Change for Children and Sure Start children's centres

A far-reaching and important document introduced by the Labour government. Published in 2003 as a Green Paper, and followed by the Children Act in 2004. *Every Child Matters* (ECM) set out the core framework for reform of children's services and aimed to improve the wellbeing of children from birth to age 19 by ensuring all organisations and workers that provide services to children, such as schools, social workers, police and health professionals, worked together in a more effective way. This multi-agency approach placed the child at the centre of everyone's attention.

The then government's aim was for every child, from birth to age 19, whatever their background or their circumstances to have the support they need to:

- Be healthy
- Stay safe
- Enjoy and achieve
- Make a positive contribution
- Achieve economic well-being (Department for Education, 2003)

(Continued)

(Continued)

2003

Sure Start children's centres

As a result of the *Every Child Matters* reform, over 3500 Sure Start children's centres were created which provide integrated services for children and their families. In 2011 the coalition government set out the following goals for children's centres in a consultation document entitled *The Core Purpose of Children's Centres*:

- *Child development and school readiness:* supporting communication, emotional, physical and social development so children start school confident and able to learn.
- *Parenting aspirations and parenting skills:* helping parents to maximise their skills and give their children the best start.
- *Child and family health and life chances*: promoting good physical and mental health for children and their parents, including addressing risk factors early on. (Department for Education, 2011d)

2004

The National Service Framework (NSF) for Children, Young People and Maternity Services

The children's NSF is aimed at all services that come into contact with children, young people or pregnant women and results in services being designed and delivered around the needs of children and families.

The NSF ensured that the *Every Child Matters* programme was delivered effectively and comprehensively. It is divided into three parts:

In Part 1, there are five standards which cover services for all children, young people and parents or carers:

- *Standard 1:* promoting health and wellbeing, identifying needs and intervening early
- *Standard 2:* supporting parenting
- *Standard 3:* child, young person and family-centred services
- *Standard 4:* growing up into adulthood
- *Standard 5:* safeguarding and promoting the welfare and children and young people.

In Part 2, there are five standards which cover services for children and young people who need specialist care, treatment or support:

- *Standard 6:* children and young people who are ill
- *Standard 7:* children in hospital

- *Standard 8:* disabled children and young people and those with complex health needs
- *Standard 9:* the mental health and psychological wellbeing of children and young people
- *Standard 10:* medicines for children and young people.

Part 3 sets out the standard for women expecting a baby and their partners and families, and for new parents:

- *Standard 11:* maternity services.

(Department of Health and Department for Education, 2004)

2005

The Social and Emotional Aspects of Learning (SEAL)

2005 saw the introduction of the Social and Emotional Aspects of Learning (SEAL) programme in primary schools with materials for secondary schools becoming available in 2007. It is a curriculum resource which aims to develop the qualities and skills required to help promote positive behaviour and effective learning. It focuses on five social and emotional aspects of learning:

- Self-awareness
- Managing feelings
- Motivation
- Empathy
- Social skills (Department for Education and Skills, 2005).

2009

The Healthy Child Programme (HCP): Pregnancy and the First Five Years of Life

The HCP aims to provide more detail on the programme that was set out in the *National Service Framework for Children, Young People and Maternity Services*. It offers every family a programme of screening tests, immunisations, developmental reviews, and information and guidance to support parenting and healthy choices – all services that children and families need to receive if they are to achieve their optimum health and wellbeing. It focuses specifically on promoting a strong parent–child attachment and positive parenting:

> The HCP is the early intervention and prevention public health programme that lies at the heart of our universal service for children and families. At a crucial stage of life, the HCP's universal reach provides an invaluable opportunity to

(Continued)

(Continued)

identify families that are in need of additional support and children who are at risk of poor outcomes. (Department of Health, 2009)

2011

Targeted Mental Health in Schools (TaMHS)

The TaMHS initial pilot programme was developed to improve the psychological well-being and mental health of children, young people and their families. The aim was that TaMHS would help schools deliver timely interventions and approaches in response to local need that could help those with mental health problems and those at increased risk of developing them (Department for Education, 2011b).

No Health Without Mental Health: A Cross-government Outcomes Strategy for People of All Ages

This strategy aims to improve mental health in all ages, and people from all backgrounds. It has six objectives:

1. More people will have good mental health
2. More people with mental health problems will recover
3. More people with mental health problems will have good physical health
4. More people will have a positive experience of care and support
5. Fewer people will suffer avoidable harm
6. Fewer people will experience stigma and discrimination (Department of Health, 2011a).

Supporting Families in the Foundation Years

In 2011 the coalition government set out its vision for the services that should be on offer for parents, children and families in the foundation years. Supporting Families in the Foundation Years describes the system needed to make the government's vision a reality and explains the role of commissioners, leaders and practitioners across the range of services for families in these years (Department for Education, 2011a).

2012

Children and Young People's Improving Access to Psychological Therapies (CYP IAPT)

In 2012 the coalition government announced that up to £32 million would be allocated to improving access to psychological therapies for children and young people in England. The

funding will provide additional training for staff and service managers in child and adolescent mental health services and ensure that more professionals are trained to deliver
appropriate, evidence-based therapies to children and young people. In the first phase, in
certain areas of the country, it has enabled more access to cognitive behavioural therapy
trained practitioners. In the second phase, it will expand to more areas and will offer systemic family therapy and interpersonal psychotherapy to help children and young people
to address problems like eating disorders, depression, self-harm and conduct problems.
The third phase will develop new e-learning tools, so staff in all sorts of settings, from GP
surgeries and schools to faith centres and police stations, can get better at working with
children and young people with mental health problems (CYP IAPT, 2013).

MENTAL HEALTH PROMOTION STRATEGIES AND PROGRAMMES

The next section of this chapter will look at some strategies and programmes that
promote the mental health of children and adolescents at different life stages. It is
clear there are critical stages in the development of a young person which involve
important transitions during which a child is more vulnerable to adversity both
within and outside the home (Loh and Wragg, 2004).

These are:

- Infancy: birth–2 years
- Early childhood: 2–5 years
- Middle childhood: 6–11 years
- Adolescence: 12–18 years.

INFANCY

Pregnancy and the first years of life are one of the most important stages of life during which the foundations of physical and mental health are laid down. The health
and wellbeing of women before, during and after pregnancy is a critical factor in
giving children a healthy start in life and laying the groundwork for good health and
wellbeing in later life. Improving maternal mental health could lead to better outcomes in childhood. Maternal depression and anxiety in pregnancy and during a
child's early life affects about 10–15% of pregnant women (O'Hara and Swain,
1996). Rates are nearly twice as high among mothers living in poverty and three
times as high for teenage mothers, and are associated with low birth weight, emotional or conduct disorders and children's later intellectual development (Hay et al.,
2001). The NSPCC report *All Babies Count* emphasises the importance of early
intervention during pregnancy and the first year, describing pregnancy as the 'magic
moment' when parents are most open to accepting help and support. It calls for
babies under 12 months who experience abuse and neglect as a result of parental

mental illness, substance misuse and domestic abuse to be the priority for services offering early intervention and involved with child protection (Cuthbert et al., 2011). The report recognises that universal services such as health visitors, children's centres and antenatal education programmes play a critical role in health care and promotion and in the early identification of families in need of additional support.

Attachment theory in particular helps to guide health professionals who are concerned with promoting mental health (Bailham and Brinley Harper, 2004). Babies and children with a secure attachment are more able to form positive relationships with care givers and others in later years. They also develop better problem solving skills, increased cooperation and are more able to show and share emotions (Dogra et al., 2002). Babies are less likely to form a secure attachment with a care giver who is stressed or depressed or unable to provide the responsive, empathic, consistent care that they need. Programmes that support parents during pregnancy and the first few years by promoting a secure attachment and addressing their mental health and emotional wellbeing are particularly important.

Activity

The guide entitled *Getting Maternity Services Right for Pregnant Teenagers and Young Fathers* (Department for Children, Schools and Families, 2008) states that teenage mothers 'are three times more likely than older mothers to develop postnatal depression, with around 40 per cent of young mothers affected'. What do you think the challenges are for teenage parents when they have a baby and think about the reasons why teenage parents are less likely to access the support of antenatal and postnatal groups.

Midwives and health visitors

There are a number of programmes aimed at supporting parents to be and reducing maternal depression. Home visiting by health visitors and midwives, which is a universal service, ensures that all pregnant women are visited before and after the baby is born and enables health professionals to pick up on signs of postnatal depression. *No Health Without Mental Health* (Department of Health, 2011a) pledges to increase the number of health visitors by 4200. These health visitors, working with Sure Start children's centres and GPs, will pay particular attention to maternal and infant mental health.

The Family Nurse Partnership Programme

Universal services such as midwives, health visitors and children's centres are essential for all families with babies and young children and are critical in promoting mental health. For some first-time young mothers and fathers, a more intensive approach is needed. The Family Nurse Partnership is a programme based on an

American model called the Nurse–Family Partnership and has been introduced in England, Scotland and Northern Ireland. This programme works intensively with young, vulnerable families for the first two years of a baby's life offering intensive and structured home visiting, delivered by specially trained nurses.

The Family Nurse Partnership aims to improve:

- Pregnancy outcomes
- Child health and development
- Parents' economic self-sufficiency.

The methods are based on theories of human ecology, self-efficacy and attachment. Central to the approach is the quality of the relationship between the parents and the nurse which aims to foster self-esteem, tackle emotional problems and bring about behaviour change which enables the parents to cope better and respond more to the needs of their child.

The Family Nurse Partnership was piloted in 2007 and has been extended by the coalition government but is only available in some areas of England. Its long-term impact of the Family Nurse Partnership Programme in England is unknown as yet, although research evidence from three randomised control trials in the USA has shown it to have positive effects from pregnancy through to the time children are 15 years old. The findings of the research show that risk factors for the child are reduced. The mothers had fewer and more widely spaced subsequent pregnancies and experienced improved financial status. The likelihood of child abuse and accidents is reduced. The children are likely to have improved developmental outcomes as they reach school age and there is clear evidence for a reduction in antisocial behaviour in children when they reach their teens (Barnes et al., 2011).

The Solihull Approach

Looking back at Chapter 1 we know that risk factors within the family have a significant impact on the mental health of the children. Difficulties with attachment, parental mental illness, conflict, inconsistent and unclear discipline can lead to difficulties in behaviour, poor self-esteem, poor school attendance and academic failure. Strategies aimed at supporting parents, improving their self-esteem and emotional wellbeing and increasing the protective factors around the child will, in turn, promote the emotional wellbeing of the child. The Solihull Approach integrates psychodynamic and behavioural theories and is aimed at professionals working with children aged 0–5 and families affected by emotional and behavioural difficulties. The concepts of containment, reciprocity and behaviour are central to the approach.

Containment is the process by which one person is able to listen to, understand and reflect back the emotional communication of another. For example, a health visitor goes to visit a mother who is exhausted and overwhelmed by the demands of her 6-month-old baby who cries and frets and can't seem to settle. The mother is unable to meet the needs of her baby because of her exhaustion and low mood. The health visitor then responds to the mother's strong emotions in an empathic and non-judgemental way. In this way, the mother feels heard, her emotions have been 'contained' by the health visitor and so the mother is more able to 'contain' and respond to the baby's emotions.

Reciprocity describes the interactions between a parent and a child. The child signals something and the parent picks up on that signal and responds appropriately. Going back to the first example, the baby's fretfulness might be a sign that he is tired and needs to sleep. A responsive parent will pick up on the signs and put the baby in his cot for a sleep or rock him gently. Sometimes a parent who is depressed or distracted is unable to respond appropriately – they might ignore the baby or try to feed him or distract him with tickling or a loud noise. This affects the process of reciprocity and impacts on the relationship and attachment between care giver and child.

Behaviour management is inevitably affected by containment and reciprocity. A child whose emotions have not been adequately contained and who has not experienced reciprocity is more likely to have behavioural problems. By introducing relevant behaviour management strategies and appropriate boundaries a parent is using a form of containment. In turn, by understanding the reason for the behaviour and responding to that rather than using a 'one size fits all' behaviour strategy, the parent is showing reciprocity.

Using the Solihull Approach, professionals involved with families who are experiencing difficulties will listen and respond to the parent's concerns in a thoughtful and empathic way and will help them to feel more in control of their emotions. This then enables the parents to reflect on the way that they interact with their child and with the help of the professional find alternative ways of meeting their needs and managing their behaviour (Solihull NHS, 2006). The Solihull Approach has the potential of increasing protective factors for babies by addressing the emotional needs of the parent and promoting a more secure attachment. However, as with the Family Nurse Partnership, the Solihull Approach has been adopted in some areas, not universally. Professionals using the Solihull Approach with parents of toddlers and preschool children help them to encourage positive interactions with others and developing their social skills, promoting their self-esteem through positive behaviour strategies and enabling them to understand and manage difficult emotions.

Parenting programmes

Children's experience of family is a critical factor in determining their positive emotional wellbeing and a healthy self-image and sense of worth. The *Good Childhood Report* (2012) states that:

> Family is the most important component of well-being for most children. Our research shows that the quality of children's relationships with their families is far more important than the particular structure of the family that they live in. For example, levels of family harmony or conflict are strongly associated with children's overall well-being, irrespective of the type of family structure. Also, children who feel more listened to and involved in making decisions within the family have significantly higher levels of well-being. (The Children's Society, 2012: 4)

So, regardless of the family structure, positive, harmonious relationships help children's wellbeing. In many families this is more or less the norm and children experience positive parenting and develop well physically and mentally. In other families parents struggle to adapt to the changing needs of their children and experience problems which can negatively impact on the child.

Becoming a parent can be one of the most difficult transitions in any person's life. Along with the excitement and joy that a young child can bring, there are also emotional and practical upheavals that affect parents' self-esteem and increase their self-doubt. Our own experience of childhood and the parenting we experienced can often affect the way that we parent our own children. We might have an idealised image of what parenthood should feel like but often the stresses and strains of trying to live up to this image can create anxious parents who question their skills and experience a sort of paralysis when it comes to imposing boundaries.

An effective intervention to help parents develop positive parenting skills is group-based parent programmes. Studies have shown that there is an improvement in children's behaviour when parents attend group-based parenting programmes that include establishment of positive support networks and mutual learning (McGuire, 1998, cited in Waldsax, 2004; Barlow, 1999, cited in Dwivedi and Brinley Harper, 2004). There are many different parenting programmes offered by a number of agencies which aim to provide guidance and support to parents of children of all ages. In April 2012, the coalition government announced a pilot project in three areas across England which offers free universal parenting classes, face-to-face and online. The classes are designed to strengthen parenting skills, and to encourage parents to feel that it is normal to get help in the first few years of their child's life – just as they do in antenatal classes before their child is born. The providers offer a mix of classes, catered to different groups of parents, informed by evidence of what works best (Department for Education, 2012c).

A Department for Education document entitled *Finding a Parenting Programme* (2012c) lists and evaluates all of the evidence-based parenting programmes. The NICE (2006) guidelines for group-based parent training/education programmes in the management of children with conduct disorders suggest that all group-based and individual programmes should:

- Be based on principles of social learning theory which suggests that we learn by observing other people;
- Include ways of improving family relationships;
- Offer 8 to 12 sessions;
- Help parents to identify their own parenting goals;
- Include role play during sessions and homework to do between sessions so that parents can practise skills;
- Be delivered by well-trained facilitators who have access to ongoing training and who are able to help parents to bring about changes in their children;
- Follow the programme's instruction manual and use relevant resources to ensure consistency (NICE, 2006).

One of the most widely used parenting programmes used by Sure Start centres nationwide is the Incredible Years Programme developed in the USA by Carolyn Webster-Stratton (2006). This programme aims to:

- Promote positive parenting;
- Improve parent–child relationships;
- Reduce critical and physical discipline and increase the use of positive strategies;
- Help parents to identify social learning theory principles for managing behaviour;
- Improve home–school relationships.

There is also an Incredible Years parenting, baby and toddler programme which supports parents-to-be and builds optimal parenting skills. The theoretical base of this programme is social learning theory, which assumes that children's behaviour will improve if it is appropriately reinforced. So good behaviour is rewarded and bad behaviour is ignored or dealt with through the loss of privileges or through 'time out' (Webster-Stratton, 2006).

Activity

The Solihull Approach and Incredible Years are universal programmes aimed at all parents and carers. There are some vulnerable families that benefit from a more focused and structured approach. Mellow Parenting is an organisation founded in Scotland offering training to professionals working with vulnerable families. Look at their website, which can be found at www.mellowparenting.org. Read the information that is given under the heading Core Programme and make notes on how the approach differs from the more universal parenting programmes. Reflect on why these differences are important for more vulnerable families.

EARLY CHILDHOOD

The next life stage from ages 2 to 5 is when children start to separate from their care giver as they discover the wider world. In infancy the children are never far from their care givers but in toddlerhood children start to try things out on their own, they become more autonomous, which often clashes with the care giver's need to keep the child close and safe from danger. Toddlers also begin to be able to understand their own and others' emotions more, particularly the four basic emotions of sadness, happiness, anger and fear. Children of this age start to be able to regulate their emotions and are able to distinguish between their own and others' emotions. Their increased proficiency with spoken language allows them to talk about their feelings, which further increases their emotional development (Loh and Wragg, 2004). The ability to communicate emotions becomes more important in early childhood; being able to express and resolve difficult emotions aids healthy emotional and social development. Toddlers begin to socialise and learn important skills needed in friendship. Play is essential, satisfying the young child's curiosity and desire for new experiences and information. Through play children develop language, learn social skills, problem solve, release tension, express emotion and have fun.

Mental health promotion strategies aimed at this developmental stage are well placed in Early Years settings which provide children with a safe, fun environment in which they can discover new experiences and people.

Since the Child Care Act was passed in 2006, all 3- and 4-year-olds are entitled to a free nursery place until they reach compulsory school age. In September 2012, it was announced that 2-year-olds are entitled to a free place in an Early Years setting as part of the Government's Fairness Premium, to drive up social mobility and improve life chances. The primary focus will be on disadvantaged children, who are currently less likely to access the benefits of early education. The new entitlement will be implemented in two phases. In September 2013, around 130,000 (20%) 2-year-olds in England will be able to access free early education places. From 2014, the entitlement will be extended to around 260,000 (40%) 2-year-olds (Department for Education, 2012b).

Early Years settings are well placed to promote mental health strategies that promote resilience in young children and reduce risk factors, particularly for those young children from more vulnerable families where more risk factors are present. The document *Promoting Children's Mental Health in Early Years and School Settings* (2001) suggests that the following factors benefit young children in Early Years settings:

- Stable child care arrangements so that children interact with just a few primary care givers in any one day;
- Low staff turnover so that children are cared for by the same individuals over several years;
- Good staff training in child development;
- Adequate staff to child ratios;
- Positive behaviour management (Department for Education and Employment, 2001).

This document also sets out the Curriculum Guidance for the Foundation Stage in relation to children's personal, social and emotional development and directs practitioners to pay particular attention to:

- Establishing constructive relationships with children, with other practitioners, between practitioners and children, with parents and with workers from other agencies, that take account of differences and different needs and expectations;
- Planning activities that promote emotional, moral, spiritual and social development alongside intellectual development;
- Providing support and a structured approach to achieve the successful social and emotional development of vulnerable children and those with particular behavioural and communication difficulties (Department for Education and Employment, 2001).

> **Activity**
>
> From age 5 to 16 children in the UK must attend school. Education plays a huge part in promoting mental health and emotional wellbeing. Think back to your school days and write two lists. (1) The negative effects on my emotional wellbeing. (2) The positive effects on my emotional wellbeing.

MIDDLE CHILDHOOD

In the UK, the year in which children turn 5 is the year they start school and there they will stay for the next 12 or 14 years of their life. During this developmental stage children are more able to regulate and mask emotions and more complex emotions such as pride, shame and guilt begin to emerge (Eriksen, 1965). With these feelings comes the fear of failure, feelings of inadequacy and low self-esteem, or pride if they do well. Children's family, upbringing and environment have an enormous impact on their healthy emotional development and sense of self but children spend five days a week, 40 weeks a year at school. Mental health promotion programmes that are school based are well placed to improve the mental health and boost the emotional resilience of pupils (Chambers and Licence, 2004). Research has shown that programmes that take a whole school approach and involve staff and pupils over prolonged periods of time seem to improve mental health outcomes of pupils (Wells et al., 2001).

Social and Emotional Aspects of Learning

The SEAL programme was developed in 2005 and aimed to provide schools with a structured whole-curriculum framework for developing all children's social, emotional and behavioural skills. SEAL was designed to promote the development of five core emotional and social skills:

- Self-awareness
- Managing feelings
- Motivation
- Empathy
- Social skills.

It was first implemented as part of the national Behaviour and Attendance Pilot in 2003 and is currently used in more than 80% of primary schools across England. Research has shown that the primary SEAL programme had a positive impact on children's wellbeing, confidence, social and communication skills and relationships, including bullying, playtime behaviour, pro-social behaviour and attitudes towards school (Hallam et al., 2006).

SEAL is delivered in three waves (Department for Education and Skills, 2005):

Wave 1 is a whole school approach which promotes emotional health and wellbeing through lessons targeting all pupils.

Wave 2 involves small group interventions for children who are thought to require additional support to develop their social and emotional skills by:

- Facilitating their personal development;
- Exploring key issues with them in more depth;
- Allowing them to practise new skills in an environment in which they feel safe, can take risks and learn more about themselves;
- Developing ways of relating to others;
- Promoting reflection.

Research has shown that small group work has a positive impact on children's emotional development (Humphrey et al., 2008).

Wave 3 of the SEAL programme involves 1:1 intervention with children who have not benefited from the whole school and small group provision and who are experiencing mental health problems.

NURTURE GROUPS

Some children who experience more risk factors than others will find it more difficult to thrive in a school environment and benefit from small group work which focuses on building their self-esteem, confidence and social skills as well as the traditional curriculum. Nurture groups were started in East London by Marjorie Boxhall in the 1970s and 1980s:

A nurture group is a small group of 6 to 10 children / young people usually based in a mainstream educational setting and staffed by two supportive adults. Nurture groups offer a short term, focussed, intervention strategy, which addresses barriers to learning arising from social / emotional and or behavioural difficulties, in an inclusive, supportive manner. Children continue to remain part of their own class group and usually return full time within 4 terms. (Nurture Groups, n.d.)

Nurture groups are based on attachment theory and promote secure, happy relationships between pupils and staff. They are an effective, evidence-based approach enabling pupils to build trusting relationships with reliable and consistent adults and with their peer group. Positive relationships and good social skills are an important protective factor and help children to develop self-esteem. Poor relationships and poor social skills can lead to rejection and isolation. The experience of healthy, consistent relationships is at the foundation of healthy emotional development. The small group work and consistent structured approach in nurture groups help children grow in self-confidence and learn to take responsibility for their behaviour, which impacts positively on their relationships and educational development (Lucas et al., 2006).

ADOLESCENCE

From 11 to 18, young people undergo huge change both emotionally and physically and this can be one of the most difficult developmental stages to negotiate. The stereotypical image of the moody, temperamental teenager, shunning adult authority and hiding themselves away in their rooms or roaming around in a pack is familiar to all. On a physical level the teenager's body is changing quickly and the emotional impact can be huge, especially for those who mature either much earlier or much later than their peers. Cognitive development in adolescents means that they become much more aware of the views of others, particularly needing the approval of peers. This time of heightened self-consciousness can lead to feelings of isolation and anxiety. At the same time adolescents start to explore their identities and seek greater autonomy. Part of the process of searching for an individual identity involves a degree of emotional separation from parents and closer identification with peers. If young people have poor social skills and low self-esteem, it can be more difficult for them to identify with and gain the support they need from their peer group. Alongside the emotional and physical changes, adolescents start to become increasingly interested in romantic involvement and sex and these relationships impact on self-esteem and add to the confusion over identity. All these changes have the potential to create emotional distress and have an impact on mental health (Loh and Wragg, 2004).

Mental health promotion strategies are particularly important at this stage, and secondary schools are the logical place for interventions aimed at children and young people in adolescence. Greater numbers and the pressure on schools to hit targets make it more difficult to reach vulnerable young people. Secondary schools are particularly concerned with preparing young people for exams and for entering the adult world well equipped. Most schools recognise the link between emotional wellbeing and academic achievement and are supportive of strategies to improve mental health. However, they also have the potential to create an environment where achievement and exam success are paramount and teaching staff are so focused on the academic progress of a pupil that they fail to notice important signs of emotional and mental distress (Prever, 2006).

The report *What Works in Developing Children's Emotional and Social Competence and Wellbeing?* concluded that good practice in schools:

> ... fosters warm relationships, encourages participation, develops teacher and pupil autonomy, and promotes clarity about boundaries, rules and expectations. (Weare and Gray, 2003: 7)

Secondary schools need to help young people to feel supported, valued and secure, give them a sense of belonging and recognise the importance of building resilience and positive self-esteem. Universal programmes such as SEAL aim to provide whole-school approaches that involve everyone in the school including pupils, staff, families and the community, and to change the environment and culture of the school. In reality it is difficult to implement change like this because secondary schools are such large organisations that have to fulfil so many different tasks and roles. Secondary SEAL was evaluated in 2010 by the Department for Children, Schools and Families and found that the programme was less successful than in primary schools. A lack of consistent school approach as well as pressures of timing, resources and staffing made it more difficult to implement (Department for Education, 2010).

United Kingdom Resilience Programme

Building resilience is an important factor in helping pupils to cope with stress, maintain a positive sense of self and regulate emotions. Resilience research has found that protective factors are more important than risk factors and that:

> ... regardless of the type of risk factor an individual is exposed to, internal and external protective factors can mitigate the risk. (Knight, 2007, cited in Shochet et al., 2009: 23)

The United Kingdom Resilience Programme (UKRP) was designed to encourage resilience and self-esteem. It was run as a pilot project for Year 7 pupils in a number of schools in England in 2008–2009. The programme aimed to build resilience and promote realistic thinking, adaptive coping skills and social problem solving in children. The evaluation found that although it was a universal programme, the general population of Year 7 pupils did not benefit greatly over a two-year period. However, the impact of the programme was much stronger for more deprived and lower-attaining pupils and those who started the year with worse psychological health, suggesting that a targeted approach to working with more vulnerable, at risk groups would be more beneficial than a universal approach which is more inconsistent in outcomes because of problems with staffing, resourcing and levels of commitment (Department for Education, 2011c).

There are many risk factors that occur in adolescence which might make a young person more vulnerable to emotional distress. Two of those risk factors which are particularly prevalent at this stage of life are bullying and substance misuse. Both factors are issues in every secondary school and have the potential to cause and add to emotional and mental ill health. Any strategy aiming to promote mental health in adolescents has to look at tackling the causes and results of both.

Bullying

It is important to make the point that bullying is obviously not exclusive to adolescence and does not only occur in schools. Primary aged children and adults experience bullying and have to deal with its devastating effects. However, bullying in adolescence is particularly insidious because it is so easy for the bullies to remain 'under the radar' and secondary schools are so large that they find it particularly difficult to tackle bullying effectively.

Children and young people who experience bullying often manage to cope and get through the experience without too many ill effects (Prever, 2006). For some who experience severe bullying over a long period of time the outcome can be much worse. It can lead to feelings of worthlessness, loss of self-esteem, self-hatred, social isolation, anxiety and depression. Some may start to harm themselves and have thoughts of suicide and in the worst cases succeed in taking their own life.

It is not only the victims that need to be the focus of strategies to combat the effects of bullying; the perpetrators are often exposed to risk factors that have led to their harmful and antisocial behaviour. Thompson et al. (2009) list the following risk factors in both the bully and victim:

- Insecure attachment
- Harsh physical discipline
- Being the victim of overprotective parenting
- Parental maltreatment and abuse.

Preventing and Tackling Bullying is a document produced by the Department for Education (2012c) in 2012 which gives advice to head teachers, staff and governing bodies to help schools prevent and respond to bullying as part of their overall behaviour policy and to understand their legal responsibilities in this area. It outlines the government's approach to bullying, legal obligations and the powers schools have to tackle bullying, and the principles which underpin the most effective anti-bullying strategies in schools.

Section 89 of the Education and Inspections Act 2006 requires that every school encourage good behaviour and prevent all forms of bullying amongst pupils. It stated that these measures should be part of the school's behaviour policy which must be communicated to all pupils, school staff and parents.

In 2011 the Department for Education commissioned research on 'The Use and Effectiveness of Anti-bullying Strategies in Schools' undertaken by Goldsmiths, University of London with the support of the Anti-Bullying Alliance (Thompson and Smith, 2011). The report looks at a variety of approaches to tackling bullying in schools including:

- PSHE lessons
- SEAL
- The school environment
- Parental/carer involvement
- Restorative strategies
- Classroom strategies
- Curriculum work
- Circle time and quality circles
- Playground strategies.

The report found that:

- Most whole-school approaches were used by schools and generally rated as effective in embedding an anti-bullying ethos;
- Most schools used PSHE education, assemblies and SEAL, reporting them as effective, economical and easy to deliver in the prevention of bullying;
- Developing a restorative ethos and culture was seen as second only to PSHE education in reducing bullying but, as with SEAL, slightly fewer schools found them easy to implement although the percentage was still high;
- Although cost-effective, only three-quarters of schools found the National Healthy Schools Programme had an impact on bullying;
- Fewer than three-quarters of schools improved their school environment despite recognising this as effective against bullying, as it was costly and difficult to do.

Activity

Research specific anti-bullying projects that are available and used by secondary schools.

Substance misuse

Part of the adolescent's journey into adulthood involves some risk taking behaviour and experimentation with alcohol, tobacco and sometimes drugs. In British culture drinking alcohol is seen as an acceptable and regular part of adult life and not surprisingly young people will start to drink alcohol as they reject their childhood games and start to feel that they are ready to join the 'grown ups'. For many young people occasional alcohol and drug use can be seen as a rite of passage and they will not go on to develop drug- and alcohol-related problems. For others, often those who already experience other risk factors, the use of drugs and alcohol can become 'substance misuse'. Alcohol and drug misuse is stated as one of the environmental factors that affect the mental health of children and young people (Prever, 2006). Young people already suffering from mental health problems such as anxiety, depression or psychotic disorders might use drugs and alcohol as a way of self-medicating in an attempt to mask or lesson the symptoms of their mental health problem and in doing so may trigger or worsen the initial problem. Pilgrim (2009: 39) points out that mental health professionals see substance misuse as a 'free-standing mental disorder and a common presenting problem in medicine, affecting health in a variety of ways'. It is clear that strategies which aim to raise awareness of the harmful effects of alcohol and drugs and to reduce their use are essential to ensure the mental health of young people.

In 2005, Ofsted published a report looking at the effectiveness of drug education in schools and found that pupils' knowledge and understanding of drugs and their effects had improved. The more effective lessons also challenged pupils' attitudes and helped them to develop decision making skills and assertiveness (Her Majesty's Chief Inspector of Schools, 2005).

A new drug strategy launched in 2010 highlighted that education is one of the most effective ways of preventing drug and alcohol misuse. The drug strategy outlines the need for young people to have access to universal drug and alcohol education. The strategy specifically states that school staff should have the information, advice and power to:

- ... provide accurate information on drugs and alcohol via drug education as well as targeted information from the FRANK* service
- tackle problem behaviour in schools, with wider powers of search and confiscation
- work with local voluntary organisations, the police and others on prevention. (HM Government , 2010: 10)

*FRANK is a government backed organisation that provides drug information to young people and their parents and carers through their website talktofrank.com. Launched in 2003, FRANK focuses on empowering young people by giving clear, impartial information about drugs and their effects.

A survey carried out by the NHS Information Centre in 2011 showed that drug and alcohol use amongst young people has decreased in the last 10 years:

- In 2011, 17% of pupils had ever taken drugs, compared with 29% in 2001.
- The proportion of pupils who drank alcohol in the last week had fallen from 26% in 2001 to 12% in 2011.

It is very difficult to accurately assess the effectiveness of drug and alcohol awareness strategies such as media campaigns and education programmes, but the fact that drug and alcohol use among young people has decreased suggests that something is working. It is also important to point out that the number of young people successfully completing treatment in specialist substance misuse services has more than doubled in five years (National Treatment Agency for Substance Misuse, 2010).

SOCIAL MEDIA AND MENTAL HEALTH PROMOTION

It is impossible to write about the emotional wellbeing and mental health of children and young people without mentioning the huge impact of social media and social networking internet sites. The harmful and dangerous impact of cyber-bullying is a constant concern for professionals working with children. The internet is also the ideal forum for those who seek to take advantage or groom young people. There is without doubt a risk to children and young people who have 24-hour access to the internet and who are not suitably supervised or educated about the risks. However, for better or worse, we cannot escape that the internet is an integral part of our lives and is a logical way to connect with children and young people who are seeking information and advice, and sometimes a way to connect with people when they feel, for whatever reason, disconnected to those around them.

The availability of information, guidance and advice is almost limitless but also sometimes misguided and potentially harmful. For very many young people the internet will be the first place they go to for information so the potential for giving appropriate, accessible, evidence-based, useful and relevant information and guidance cannot be ignored.

In July 2013 a new online charity called MindFull was launched giving 11- to 17-year-olds immediate access to free online professional counselling support and advice. MindFull gives children and teenagers the support of mental health professionals and enables them to mentor one another in a safe space. The charity also educates young people about how to cope with mental health issues – providing information, advice and guidance, both online and through training in schools (MindFull, 2013). It important that children and young people have support through their peers and through online sites as so many are reluctant to talk to adults about their worries and find the anonymity of online support less threatening. In a survey carried out by MindFull, 57% of children said that they would prefer to confide in a friend and 68% thought that putting mental health services online would be an effective way to tackle mental health issues among young people. The online support is offered by British Association for Counselling and Psychotherapy (BACP) trained counsellors who would refer children and young people to mental health services when appropriate (MindFull, 2013).

CONCLUSION

This chapter has outlined a very small number of strategies used to promote mental health and emotional wellbeing in children and young people. As has been shown by the decreased number of young people using drugs and alcohol, strategies that inform and educate young people can be successful. Over the last few years campaigns such as Time to Change, and storylines on soaps watched by millions that represent young people with mental health problems in a responsible, relevant way are starting to diminish the stigma attached to mental ill health. This will hopefully lead to a society that is aware of the signs of mental health problems and give confidence to children, young people and their families, encouraging them to speak out and seek appropriate help and support.

REFERENCES

Bailham, D. and Brinley Harper, P. (2004) 'Attachment Theory and Mental Health'. In K. Dwivedi and P. Brinley-Harper (eds), *Promoting the Emotional Well–being of Children and Adolescents and Preventing their Mental Ill Health*. London: Jessica Kingsley, pp. 49–68.

Barnes, J., Ball, M., Meadows, P. et al. (2011) *The Family–Nurse Partnership Programme in England: First Year Pilot Sites Implementation in England. Pregnancy and the Post-partum Period.* London: Department for Children, School and Families.

CAMHS (2008) *Child and Adolescent Mental Health Services Review.* Available from: www.bacp.co.uk/admin/structure/files/pdf/11791_sbc_may2013.pdf (accessed August 2013).

Centre for Mental Health (2010) *The Economic and Social Costs of Mental Health Problems in 2009/10.* Available from: www.centreformentalhealth.org.uk/pdfs/Economic_and_social_costs_2010.pdf (accessed 19 November 2013).

Chambers, R. and Licence, K. (2004) *Looking After Children in Primary Care: A Companion to the Children's National Service Framework.* London: Radcliffe.

The Children's Society (2012) *The Good Childhood Report 2012: A Summary of our Findings.* Available at: www.childrenssociety.org.uk/what-we-do/research/well-being/good-child-hood-report-2012 (accessed 10 February 2013).

Cuthbert, C., Rayns, G. and Stanley, K. (2011) *All Babies Count: Prevention and Protection for Vulnerable Babies.* London: NSPCC. Available from: www.nspcc.org.uk/Inform/resourcesforprofessionals/underones/all_babies_count_pdf_wdf85569.pdf.

CYP IAPT (Children and Young People's Improving Access to Psychological Therapies) (2013) *Children and Young People's Briefing.* Available from: www.iapt.nhs.uk/silo/files/cyp-iapt-key-facts-july-2013-.pdf (accessed 19 November 2013).

Department for Children, Schools and Families (2008) *Getting Maternity Services Right for Pregnant Teenagers and Young Fathers.* London: DCSF.

Department for Education (2010) *Social and Emotional Aspects of Learning Programme in Secondary Schools: National Evaluation.* London: DfE.

Department for Education (2011a) *Supporting Families in the Foundation Years.* Available from: www.education.gov.uk/childrenandyoungpeople/earlylearningandchildcare/early/a00192398/supporting-families-in-the-foundation-years (accessed 23 October 2012).

Department for Education (2011b) *Targeted Mental Health in Schools.* Available from: www.education.gov.uk/publications/standard/publicationDetail/Page1/DFE-RR177 (accessed 2 October 2012).

Department for Education (2011c) *UK Resilience Programme Evaluation: Final Report.* Available from: www.education.gov.uk/publications/eOrderingDownload/DFE-RR097.pdf (accessed 26 February 2013).

Department for Education (2011d) *The Core Purpose for Sure Start Children's Centres.* Available from: www.education.gov.uk/childrenandyoungpeople/earlylearningand-childcare/a00191780/core-purpose-of-sure-start-childrens-centres (accessed 2 October 2012).

Department for Education (2012b) *Statutory Guidance for Local Authorities on the Delivery of Free Early Education for Three and Four Year Olds and Securing Sufficient Childcare.* London: DfE.

Department for Education (2012c) *Finding a Parenting Programme.* Available from: www.education.gov.uk/commissioning-toolkit (accessed 16 October 2012).

Department for Education (2012e) *Preventing and Tackling Bullying.* London: DfE. Available at: http://webarchive.nationalarchives.gov.uk/20130401151715/https://www.education.gov.uk/publications/eOrderingDownload/preventing%20and%20tackling%20bullying.pdf (accessed 19 November 2013).

Department for Education and Employment (2001) *Promoting Children's Mental Health within Early Years and School Settings.* London: DfEE.

Department for Education and Skills (2003) *Every Child Matters.* London: DfES. Available from: www.education.gov.uk/publications/standard/publicationDetail/Page1/DfES%200672%202003 (accessed 2 October 2012).

Department for Education and Skills (2005) *Excellence and Enjoyment: Social and Emotional Aspects of Learning: Guidance.* Nottingham: DfES Publications.

Department of Health and Department of Education (2004) *National Service Framework for Children, Young People and Maternity Services.* Available from: www.dh.gov.uk/en/Publicationsandstatistics/Publications/PublicationsPolicyAndGuidance/DH_4089100 (accessed 23 October 2012).

Department of Health (2009) *The Healthy Child Promotion Programme:* Available from: www.dh.gov.uk/en/Publicationsandstatistics/Publications/PublicationsPolicyAndGuidance/DH_107563 (accessed 2 October 2012).

Department of Health (2011a) *No Health without Mental Health: A Cross Government Mental Health Outcomes Strategy for People of all Ages.* Available from: www.dh.gov.uk/en/Publicationsandstatistics/Publications/PublicationsPolicyAndGuidance/DH_123766 (accessed March 2013).

Department of Health (2011b) *Healthy Lives, Healthy People.* Available from www.gov.uk/government/uploads/system/uploads/attachment_data/file/216096/dh_127424.pdf

Dogra, N. Parkin, A. Gale, F. and Frake, C. (2002) *A Multidisciplinary Handbook of Child and Adolescent Mental health for Front-line Professionals.* London: Jessica Kingsley.

Dwivedi, K. and Brinley Harper, P. (eds) (2004) *Promoting the Well-being of Children and Adolescents and Preventing their Mental Ill Health.* London: Jessica Kingsley.

Education and Inspections Act (2006) Section 89. Available from: www.legislation.gov.uk/ukpga/2006/40/pdfs/ukpga_20060040_en.pdf (accessed 10 February 2013).

Eriksen, E. (1965) *Childhood and Society.* Harmondsworth: Penguin.

Hallam, S., Rhamie, J. and Shaw, J. (2006) *Evaluation of the Primary Behaviour and Attendance Pilot.* London: DfES.

Hay, D.F., Pawlby, S., Sharp, D. et al. (2001) Intellectual Problems Shown by 11-year Old Children Whose Mothers had Postnatal Depression. *Journal of Child Psychology and Psychiatry, and Allied Disciplines*, 42 (7): 871–89.

Her Majesty's Chief Inspector of Schools (2005) *Drugs Education in Schools.* Available from: dera.ioe.ac.uk/5389/1/Drug%20education%20in%20schools%20%28PDF%20format%29.pdf. (accessed 23 October 2012).

HM Government (2010) *Drug Strategy 2010 Reducing Demand, Restricting Supply, Building Recovery: Supporting people to live a drug free life.* Available from: www.gov.uk/government/uploads/system/uploads/attachment_data/file/98026/drug-strategy-2010.pdf (accessed 25 October 2012).

Humphrey, N., Kalambouka, A., Bolton, J., Lendrum, A., Wigelsworth, M., Lennie, C. and Farrell, P. (2008) *Primary Social and Emotional Aspects of Learning: Small Group Work Evaluation.* Manchester: School of Education, University of Manchester.

Kim-Cohen, J., Caspi, A., Moffitt, T.E., Harrington, H., Milne, B.J. and Poulton, R. (2003) Prior Juvenile Diagnoses in Adults with Mental Disorder: Developmental Follow-back of a Prospective Longitudinal Cohort. *Archives of General Psychiatry*, 60: 709–17.

Loh, E. and Wragg, J. (2004) Developmental Perspective. In K. Dwivedi and P. Brinley-Harper (eds), *Promoting the Well–being of Children and Adolescents and Preventing their Mental Ill Health.* London: Jessica Kingsley, pp. 29–48.

Lucas, S., Insley, K. and Buckland, G. (2006) *Nurture Group Principles and Curriculum Guidelines Helping Children to Achieve.* London: The Nurture Group Network.

Mellow Parenting (n.d.) Available from: http://mellowparenting.org/ (accessed on 23 October 2012).

Mind (n.d.) Available from: www.mind.org.uk (accessed on 9 October 2012).

MindFull (2013) Available from: www.mindfull.org/static/mf/pdfs/2013_06_05.pdf?245411050713 (accessed 10 July 2013).

National Treatment Agency for Substance Misuse (2010) *Substance Misuse Among Young People: The Data 2009–2010*. NHS. Available from: www.education.gov.uk/childrenandyoungpeople/healthandwellbeing/substancemisuse/a0070053/drugs (accessed 23 October 2012).

NICE (2006) *Parent Training Programmes in the Management of Conduct Disorders*. Available from: publications.nice.org.uk/parent-trainingeducation-programmes-in-the-management-of-children-with-conduct-disorders-ta102 (accessed 13 November 2012).

Nurture Groups (n.d.) Available from: www.nurturegroups.org/ (accessed 9 October 2012).

O'Hara, M.W. and Swain, A.M. (1996) Rates and Risk of Postpartum Depression: A Meta-analysis. *International Review of Psychiatry*, 8 (1): 37–54.

Pilgrim, D. (2009) *Key Concepts in Mental Health*, 2nd edn. London: Sage.

Prever, M. (2006) M*ental Health in Schools A Guide to Pastoral and Curriculum Provision*. London: Sage.

Rethink Mental Illness (n.d.) Available from: www.rethink.org (accessed 9 October 2012).

Shochet, I., Hoge, R. and Wurfl, A. (2009) Building Resilience to Prevent Mental Health Problems in Young People: The Resourceful Adolescent Programme (RAP). In Geldard, K. (ed.) *Practical Interventions for Young People at Risk*. London: Sage pp. 22–32.

Solihull NHS Care Trust, Birmingham City University (2006) *Solihull Approach Resource Pack*, 5th edn. Cambridge: Jill Rogers Associates Ltd.

Thompson, F. and Smith, P. (2011) *The Use and Effectiveness of Anti-Bullying Strategies in Schools*. London: Department for Education.

Thompson, F. Tippett, N. and Smith. P. (2009) Prevention and Responses to Bullying. In K. Geldard (ed.) *Practical Interventions for Young People at Risk*. London: Sage pp. 90–101.

Time to Change (2012) Available from: www.time-to-change.org.uk (accessed 16 February 2012).

Waldsax, A. (2004) Parenting. In Dwivedi, K. and Brinley Harper, P. (eds) *Promoting the Well-being of Children and Adolescents and Preventing their Mental Ill Health*. London: Jessica Kingsley, pp. 113–132.

Weare, K. and Gray, G. (2003) *What Works in Developing Children's Emotional and Social Competence and Wellbeing?* Southampton: The Health Education Unit Research and Graduate School of Education, University of Southampton.

Webster-Stratton, C. (2006) *The Incredible Years*. USA: The Incredible Years.

Wells, J., Barlow, J. and Stewart-Brown, S. (2001) *A Systematic Review of Universal Approaches to Mental Health Promotion in Schools*. Oxford: Health Services Research Unit, University of Oxford.

5

EFFECTIVE COMMUNICATION WITH CHILDREN, YOUNG PEOPLE AND THEIR FAMILIES

ERICA PAVORD

> ### Overview
>
> - Verbal, non-verbal and paralinguistic communication
> - The importance of self-awareness and reflective practice
> - Therapeutic communication
> - Rogers' core conditions and the person-centred approach
> - Active listening skills
> - Blocks and barriers to effective communication

INTRODUCTION

Practitioners working with children, young people and their families or carers require good interpersonal and communication skills. Active listening skills are essential to building a therapeutic relationship. These skills are also important to the inter-professional communication between practitioners from health, social care, informal and voluntary agencies and are essential for productive teamwork and effective delivery of services. This chapter provides an opportunity to explore both the theory and practice of effective communication and the components of a therapeutic relationship and offers the opportunity to reflect on and explore the self in relation to others.

THE IMPORTANCE OF EFFECTIVE COMMUNICATION

When working with children and young people in any setting, successful communication is essential. However detailed and focused any intervention might be, it is unlikely to work if the professional involved cannot communicate effectively. Whether in a school, hospital, youth centre or in specific mental health settings, professionals will have to work with people of all ages, people with emotional and physical needs and people from diverse cultures and backgrounds. Communicating with a very angry 11-year-old boy who lashes out at anyone who challenges him or with a 15-year-old bereaved girl who is depressed may require different approaches and skills but whatever the situation and wherever the setting, the key to successful effective communication is the relationship itself. Your greatest asset when working with young people is yourself and your ability to connect with another individual and to show them that you value and respect them (Prever, 2011).

If you think back over your life to the people who have respected and connected with you, it is possible that this was because they really listened to you. At the core of effective communication is effective listening (Adler et al., 2007). The emphasis throughout this chapter is on how to show the children and young people you are working with that they have been heard and are respected. If we really listen to the children and young people that we work with and show them that we believe in them, they are more likely to feel that their feelings and thoughts are valued and this can empower them to make choices that will benefit them (McLeod, 2008).

WHAT IS COMMUNICATION?

- Communication is a process in which individuals interact with and through symbols to create and interpret meaning (Wood, 2004).
- Any interaction that takes place between people (Donnelly and Neville, 2008).

It is clear from these definitions that communication is not solely reliant on speech but on a complex interplay of language, gesture and facial expression. It is further influenced by the context of both the environment and the culture of the people involved in the interaction.

Different kinds of communication

It is important to be able to distinguish between the different kinds of communication and to understand how each will affect the interaction between two or more people.

There are three main kinds of communication to consider:

- *Interpersonal communication:* that which takes place between people.
- *Environmental communication:* that which takes place within our environment.
- *Intra-personal communication:* that which takes place within ourselves (Donnelly and Neville, 2008).

To illustrate how the different kinds of communication interact with each other, imagine this, not uncommon, scenario. In a secondary school, a teenage boy who has had very little sleep because he has been up half the night after an argument with his dad, is found wandering around the corridors during lesson time by a teacher. The teacher, who has just had a really difficult lesson, immediately shouts at the boy and orders him back to his lesson. The boy swears at the teacher and runs off. It is clear that the interpersonal communication has been very unsuccessful because each participant's internal thoughts and feelings have collided in an environment that is not conducive to a warm chat. Think now about how much more effective this communication could have been. The teacher sees the boy, asks him if he needs any help. The boy explains why he's late, and the teacher suggests they have a chat in his office/classroom. They sit down and the boy talks a bit about the night before. The teacher listens and the boy feels heard and supported. This example is a simple illustration of how ineffective communication can cause so many problems in families, schools and workplaces (Adler et al., 2007). It is so important to consider the context of the child or young person and to be aware of what they might be going through and how their experiences affect their ability to cope in day-to-day situations.

INTERPERSONAL COMMUNICATION

There are three main kinds of interpersonal communication which react together to create a particular kind of interaction:

- Verbal
- Non-verbal
- Paralinguistic.

Verbal

We do not need words to communicate; our facial expressions, body language, gestures communicate a huge amount. From the beginning of life we are communicating. Babies in a supportive environment usually manage to get their needs met within a sensitive nurturing reciprocal relationship without any spoken words but they generally develop the ability to speak by the age of 3 because language is so central to our existence as relational human beings. Adler et al. (2007: 114) suggest that 'without the ability to use language we would hardly be human – at least not in the usual sense of the word'. So language, whether it be spoken or signed, is the vehicle for allowing us to express who we are and how we relate to those around us.

However, the way that we use language, our verbal communication, can be complex. When considering the importance of verbal communication with children and young people with mental health issues we need to be aware of the impact of our choice of language on them. Words and phrases can have an explicit or surface meaning, and an implicit or hidden meaning. Think, for example of the many different ways we can say the simple word 'hello' and the many interpretations that can be made. 'Hello' can be said in so many ways: friendly, suspicious, sarcastic, suggestive, questioning ... and many more. The relationships that you will have with the children or young people in the work setting will involve much more complex communication and so it is essential to remember that the context of the words spoken can depend on many different things; the way they are said, where they are said, who says them and who hears them. Language is subjective and people may attach different meanings to the same message depending on their experience, environment, age, gender, culture; even on what might have happened to them five minutes ago (Adler et al., 2007).

The meaning of words alters greatly between different generations, cultures and regions. Think of the language of a typical adolescent of 2014 and how that compares with a 70-year-old. Many words have changed their meaning over the years – 'gay', 'cool', for instance. As an older person working with a teenager we can often feel our age when they talk to us in the language of their peers. Geldard and Geldard (2010) suggest that it is preferable to be honest and ask the young person directly what the word means. In my experience, teenagers do not expect me to understand some of the language they use and are pleased to explain – it can often help the relationship and the power balance to be the person who doesn't understand and for the young person to be the one with the knowledge.

It is also important to consider how our language might be understood by someone with English as an additional language. Think of a 10-year-old asylum seeker whose English might be good enough to cope in a classroom situation with teaching assistants and written visual aids to assist him but who finds the nuances of language heard in the playground far too subtle and might frequently get the wrong end of the stick. Think too of a child on the autistic spectrum who will understand what is said literally and might act on it. People with autism have a very literal understanding of language and often don't understand common phrases (National Autistic Society, 2012). A good example of this is a carer working with an autistic 17-year-old boy. She was busy helping someone else when he asked for her help. She told him to 'hold on' and was then surprised to find him holding on to the sleeve of her cardigan.

Paralinguistic

Paralinguistic communication refers to the different way we might moderate our speech according to the situation. The pitch, tone, volume, rhythm and timing as well as grunts, ahs, ums can greatly affect how verbal communication might be perceived. Hargie (2011: 81) says, 'How information is delivered paralinguistically has important consequences for how much of the message is understood, recalled and acted on.' Often there is a mismatch between the words spoken and the way they are spoken and this can tell us a lot about the speaker's real meaning. For example, a teaching assistant supporting a child with acute anxiety might tell the child that it's ok if she can't cope with going to the dinner hall but uses an abrupt and impatient tone. The message the child receives is more likely to be: 'I'm so irritated with you at the moment and wish you'd make an effort'. Awareness of what message our tone is communicating can help us to avoid difficult situations. It's also essential for us as professionals to listen to the child's paralinguistic communication. We might hear them say that they had a really good time at the weekend but their tone is flat. Quite often children feel that they have to show us that things are better than they really are. They might want us to believe that the work we are doing with them is helping and so present a sunnier picture to us than the reality. Being aware of the mismatch between word and tone is very important (Culley and Bond, 2004).

Non-verbal

Non-verbal communication is visual rather than linguistic and can often be more effective than words alone. 'Non-verbal communication contributes a great deal to shaping perceptions' (Adler et al., 2007: 147). As helpers we have to be aware of what message our non-verbal communication is conveying. At the very least, it should show that we are listening (Geldard and Geldard, 2010).

Eye contact, body language, facial expressions, gestures, interpersonal space, touch and smell are all important ways of communicating meaning and can completely change the impact of words if the two are at odds with one another. It is essential to be aware of the non-verbal communication of the children and young people we work with as it often gives us more information than the words they use, particularly when the child is in distress and is unable to find the words to express themselves or in some cases, fearful of using words. A child who is using plenty of spoken language to communicate but who is unable to make eye contact might be communicating to us that what they are actually saying isn't what they want to say. A 14-year-old girl who reassures us that everything is fine at home but who is tugging on the sleeves of her jumper or keeping her hands firmly under her legs might be communicating that in fact she is very anxious or unhappy about what she is experiencing.

It is important to be aware of how different cultures might interpret body language (Koprowska, 2010). There are some non-verbal behaviours that are universal, like smiling, laughing, frowning, but different cultures have different non-verbal languages as well as verbal ones. Some cultures are openly affectionate and others less so. In France it is perfectly normal for people of all ages to 'faire la bise' – kissing on both cheeks – even when you are meeting someone for the first time. In some cultures men hold hands as a sign of solidarity or kinship and in others it will be assumed that they are gay (Khuri, 2000). The level of eye contact is very different in different cultures; staring is seen as far more acceptable in some cultures than it is in British culture. When working with children or young people from a culture different to your own it is important to be aware of potential differences and not jump to conclusions about what a look or a gesture might mean.

ENVIRONMENTAL COMMUNICATION

It is extremely important to consider the environment in which we communicate and how it might affect an interaction. A helper working in a health setting might have to see children or young people in quite clinical settings such as a consulting room in a hospital which can be intimidating and sometimes frightening. In education settings the rooms are usually set up to support teaching and learning. In a classroom setting it would be much better to sit beside a child rather than behind a teacher's desk which communicates authority. To try to communicate with an angry child across the classroom, surrounded by other children, would be far more difficult than if you were able to ask them to come out of the classroom with you, which would help to defuse the situation rather than ignite it. In specific CAMHS settings it is even more important that the environment communicates a warm and welcoming message as the children or young people attending are more likely to be anxious about being there.

Activity

Think about how the following environments communicate with the people in them. How might they help or hinder effective communication?

- The quiet area in a play group
- A busy primary school playground
- The canteen of a large secondary school
- The head teacher's office
- A psychologist's office in a hospital

Now think about your workplace. Which areas hinder communication and which areas help it?

INTRA-PERSONAL COMMUNICATION

On a simple level, intra-personal communication might be the argument we have with ourselves when we know we should tidy up the house but really want to sit and watch daytime TV.

I deserve this, I worked hard all week and the housework can wait.

You said that last week and it still isn't done.

On a deeper level, it is more complicated than that. The internal workings of our minds are complex and much of the time we might be completely unaware of the inner discourse that goes on when we are interacting with others. We all come to every relationship with our own thoughts, feelings, beliefs, values and experiences and every interaction we have will be determined by what is going on for us internally. We have looked at child development and understand that we have an internal world created according to external experiences which subsequently affects the meanings that we make of the external world. What might be an exciting experience for one person could be terrifying for another and this will affect the way that information is given and received surrounding that experience. It is essential to be aware of how our internal world might be influencing our interactions with others and, in turn, be aware of how their internal world is affecting how they are interacting with us. An example of this might be in a children's ward in a hospital. You might be a student nurse who was admitted to hospital as a child and have vivid memories of feeling frightened and alone. In your interactions with a young child and her mother you find it hard to keep your emotions in check as you assume that the child will be feeling exactly the same as you did, you might also feel judgemental towards the mother when she goes home, leaving the child alone. The intra-personal communication – 'this child is lonely and her mother is neglectful' – is probably based more on your experiences rather than theirs and might influence the way that you communicate verbally and non-verbally to them. Chapter 8 will encourage further reflection on how our beliefs and experiences affect our interactions with children and young people.

SELF-AWARENESS

In order to be able to form good relationships with children, young people and their families we need to be self-aware and able to recognise our strengths and weaknesses. Being clear and honest about our abilities and skills and our needs is important as it enables us to work professionally and with integrity. Prever (2011: 168) recognises the 'potential dangers of over-identification; the playing out of adult–child roles including issues around power; and the need to care for and protect, particularly as if in a parent role'.

Working with young people who have specific emotional needs and whose behaviour is challenging can be difficult and emotionally draining. It is not surprising that we get deeply involved with a young person's pain and suffering and professional boundaries become blurred. It can be difficult sometimes to differentiate between our own issues and those of the children and young people. For example, a mother of two who is going through a difficult divorce would need to be very careful of what and how she communicates with a young boy who is experiencing severe anxiety following the break-up of his parents' marriage. It is possible that the worker might confuse the child's feelings and experiences with those of her own children. This could lead to the worker not listening fully to the child and to him feeling unheard and unsupported. It is therefore very important that we develop ways to increase our self-awareness:

- Keep a reflective journal in which you write down your thoughts and feelings in relation to the young people you work with.
- Speak to a mentor or supervisor about the work you do and the difficulties you are facing.
- Seek open and honest feedback about the way that you work with children and young people.
- Welcome opportunities for others to observe the work that you do.
- Use a reflective tool like Gibbs to help you to reflect on a particular experience or the SWOB analysis to focus on your strengths and weaknesses.

Activity

Think back to the last time that you successfully tackled an issue you were anxious about. Reflect over the stages of what happened and what you did. What were the things that made the incident successful? What from these would you use again in similar circumstances? How did resolving this incident make you feel? Did you find that after it was resolved the incident held less importance or significance for you?

Now think of an incident where you did not follow through on the course of action that you had decided was needed. Why did you decide not to act? How satisfied are you with the outcome? Do you still find that you still think about the incident in a negative way? What do you think about it now? Is it still unfinished business?

The Gibbs reflective cycle (Gibbs, 1988)

This model of reflection (Figure 5.1) encourages you to reflect on a specific interaction and is a good way of encouraging your to reflect critically on your skills and to think of ways in which you can improve your practice.

THERAPEUTIC COMMUNICATION

In some of the interactions we have with a child or young person, it will be enough that we think sensitively about the way we communicate with them, but there may be times when we meet children who are experiencing difficulties, who are going through periods of psychological distress and are confused, angry and afraid. In

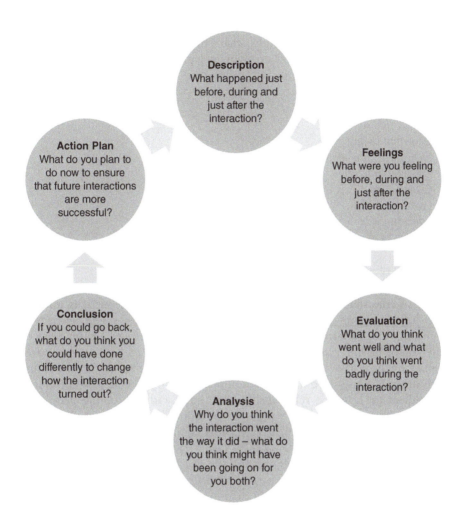

Figure 5.1 Reflecting on an interaction

Adapted from Gibbs (1988)

these cases it is important to ensure that we are not only sensitive but that we communicate with them in a therapeutic way, that we show them that we are willing to spend time getting to know them and 'walking alongside them' as they struggle to make sense of their experiences.

We have established that communication is any kind of interaction between people. If that communication is to be therapeutic it has to be of benefit to the child or young person, it has to contribute to their sense of wellbeing, and it should promote their emotional growth and development.

So much of our communication with others is non-therapeutic, whether it be intentional or not, we often end up giving negative or mixed messages, being critical or making fun of, showing our lack of interest or curiosity in the person and their concerns. Think about a 13-year-old girl's average day at school. It is very likely that she will be:

- Told what to do
- Shouted at, individually or in a group
- Given information
- Given advice
- Criticised
- Made fun of
- Addressed as part of a group rather than as an individual
- Ignored
- Patronised.

It is also true that she might be praised and encouraged but it is unlikely, even with loving, caring parents, friends and teachers, that she will be truly listened to for any more than an hour or two at best. As someone working with children and young people, you have the potential to connect with them and have an impact on how they are experiencing life through the way you communicate with them. It is useful to have a grounding of theory to enable you to understand and reflect on how the relationships you have with the young people can help them to grow in confidence and self-esteem. There are many theories which relate to working therapeutically and this chapter will focus on person-centred theory.

Carl Rogers was a psychologist and therapist working in America in the latter half of the 20th century and was the founder of client-centred therapy (Casemore, 2006). He believed passionately in the importance of listening to patients' experiences and developing a trusting relationship with them which would enable them to grow and cope with their difficulties and function more effectively. Rogers (1951) suggests that that there are three core conditions required in a therapeutic relationship:

Unconditional positive regard: the helper accepts and values the client with warmth and without judgement. The feeling of being judged is very strong in young people, particularly adolescents who are experiencing such huge physiological and emotional changes and who are struggling to find their individuality at home, at school and with their friendship groups. It is natural to put up barriers when we feel we are judged and to hide our feelings or deny them altogether. The experience of talking to someone who doesn't judge us can be very powerful and can enable us, in time, to allow ourselves to feel difficult, uncomfortable and sometimes frightening feelings which we keep hidden. Younger children are constantly being judged and told what to do and how to do things, and learn from an early age that some feelings, like happiness, are acceptable and others, like anger, are not. For them, the experience of being able to express their thoughts and feelings without being told they are wrong can be empowering. Rogers (1967: 283) says that unconditional positive regard 'involves an acceptance of and caring for the client as a "separate" person, with permission for him to have his own feelings and experiences, and to find his own meanings in them'.

Empathy: having an empathic understanding of the clients' internal reference. To have empathy for someone is the willingness to understand what it might be like to live in their shoes. To walk alongside someone and have a strong sense of how they experience life. It is not sympathy and it is not saying that you know what they are going through because you've been through it too. It is a willingness to understand their own unique experiences and feelings and to be able to reflect that understanding back to them so that they feel understood. Prever (2011: 118) says that empathy 'allows us to enter freely into the young person's often complicated, fragile, confusing and sometimes traumatic world. Empathy shows respect for, and validates, not only the child's world but the young person themselves.'

Congruence: the helper is genuine, honest and true. Children and young people seem to have an uncanny knack of knowing exactly when an adult is putting on a front and trying to be someone they are not. To be congruent with someone is to be completely honest and without pretence. It is important when listening to someone who is full of difficult feelings, who is confused and has learnt to defend themselves against painful feelings, that we be as open as possible. We need to be able to respond to the children and young people in our care in an honest and real way. It is true that sometimes there seems to be a contradiction between being non-judgemental and being congruent. We might be working with a young person who is a bully, who has intentionally hurt other, less powerful children and who we feel negative feelings towards. We might be talking to someone who has very prejudiced views that make us feel very uncomfortable. How do can we be honest and true when our feelings are negative and we want to show our disapproval of their views and actions? It is important to be able to separate the individual from their views and actions. Imagine talking to a boy who has terrorised and hurt a younger child. We can say, 'I feel really uncomfortable about what you did to that boy yesterday and I can't help thinking how scared he must have been and I'm wondering how you felt about it. What was going on for you?' This response is non-judgemental and honest.

It is certainly true that the core conditions must be at the foundation of a therapeutic relationship but it can be argued that it is not enough and that the young people in our care might need us to be more directive with them. It might also be the case that our role is to give guidance and information to help them to make good choices. Whatever our role is, it is always necessary to keep empathy, unconditional positive regard and congruence or genuineness at the core of our interactions and to remember that the relationships that we build with the young people can in themselves be a catalyst for change.

THERAPEUTIC COMMUNICATION THROUGH ACTIVE LISTENING

When we are with a young person who is experiencing emotional and mental health difficulties, how do we actually ensure that we are offering them the possibility of having a genuine, non-judgemental and empathic relationship with us where their feelings and thoughts are taken seriously and understood?

In order to address the different communication styles of different age groups, we will look first of all at communication with older children and adolescents. Here it is assumed that they will be more familiar and comfortable with the idea of talking to an adult at a certain depth. The second section will focus on more creative methods of communicating with younger children. These ideas come from play therapy and involve much more listening and observing rather than direct interventions. However, it is important to realise that older children too might find it far easier to express themselves through more creative methods like sand, paint and role play. It is equally true that a 4- or 5-year-old might have perfectly good language skills and find it easy to talk to an adult about their feelings.

Active listening with older children and adolescents

Most of us know what it's like not to be listened to. The following activity invites you to reflect on how this makes you feel.

Activity

Work with someone. Ask the other person to tell you about an experience they have just had that might be something that was annoying or frustrating. While they are speaking you must look down or look away and give them no non-verbal indicators that you are listening. When you have finished this, swap roles then discuss what it felt like to tell someone about your experience.

This activity might have felt forced and unreal but will have hopefully shown you the importance of active listening. When listening, your partner would have heard every word you said and it might well have had a significant impact on them but as a speaker you would probably have been left feeling like no one had been there at all. It is likely that most people who experience someone not listening to them are left feeling unimportant, invisible, angry and worthless. In order to show that we are empathic, non-judgemental and genuine we need to use active listening skills (Geldard and Geldard, 2010).

Eye contact

The generally accepted rule for effective active listening is that we need to maintain good eye contact. This does not mean looking into the young person's eyes all the time but it is important, especially when speaking, to have good eye contact. When listening, it often feels more natural to maintain eye contact most of the time, but to avoid making the young person feel overly scrutinised we should break eye contact momentarily. Think about the amount of eye contact you would naturally have when talking to a friend or someone you feel comfortable with. It is natural to look to the side of their face or just over their head for a second or two. Sometimes you might feel that the young person you are talking to does not make eye contact at all. They might look down or in completely the opposite direction. This could be a sign that the young person finds it difficult to communicate and feels very uncomfortable talking at any length or depth with another person, especially an adult. Sometimes a person's low self-esteem can make it feel almost impossible to maintain eye contact.

The young person might be experiencing feelings of worthlessness, which make it hard to accept that another person is taking an interest in them. It is important not to increase their discomfort by making constant eye contact but to settle on what feels comfortable whilst still letting them know that you are listening closely. Argyll (1988) suggests that breaking eye contact can help if the speaker is feeling uncomfortable.

Body language

Our body language is very important and can tell us a lot about what is going on for a young person. It is equally important for us to be aware of our own body language and think about what messages it is sending to the young person we are talking to. We should try to maintain an open posture (Culley and Bond, 2004). Crossed arms and legs can suggest that you are closed off to the person you are talking to. If the young person is sitting, it is important for you to be sitting too. You need to look relaxed, and your body should be angled towards the person, giving them enough personal space but being close enough to show you are listening to them attentively. If you are sitting, your chairs should be angled towards each other rather than squarely opposite as that could feel like an interrogation. Sometimes I will sit at a table alongside the young person I am talking to because we are drawing or looking at pictures and that feels very relaxed because there is not so much pressure to speak. If the young person needs space to think, it can feel easier if you are side by side, engaged in another activity so the pressure is off. It is sometimes best with eye contact and body language to try to mirror the person you are talking to whilst encouraging openness. If the young person is sitting almost horizontally in the chair, head back, needing to relax and think, it is more appropriate to relax back in your chair too.

Acknowledging and reflecting feeling

Feelings and emotions are words that are often used synonymously but it might be useful to distinguish between the two. Feltham and Dyrden (1993) suggest that feelings are experienced and emotions are exhibited. This can make it difficult to recognise the feeling that a young person is experiencing. They might be exhibiting an emotion of anger but actually experiencing intense sadness. It is so important for a young person to feel that they have been listened to and understood, that their feelings have been acknowledged and that their thoughts and worries are valued but this can be hard to do if the emotions they are showing are hiding the true feelings.

Sometimes our feelings are straightforward and it is easy to know when someone is angry or sad, happy or afraid. For example, a teenage girl is forbidden from going out for a week. She is really angry so she shouts at her mum, slams the door, refuses to speak for a day and shouts about how she hates her family. There is action and movement in this anger, she expresses it and processes it. Sometimes our feelings are more confused. Imagine a similar scenario but this time the feelings are confused by the difficult relationship between the girl and her mother. The girl is forbidden from going out but as well as that, her mother is aggressive and hits her. She is scared and retreats, taking the punishment silently. Here the feelings of anger and fear are confused and cause the girl to remain static, unable to process her feelings. She might not show any emotion at all, so for an outsider it can be difficult to know in a situation like this exactly what the feelings are. The girl is not able to express them so she has to keep them hidden. She internalises her feelings. It is really important to give young people time to first understand and then work through their feelings.

Sometimes we don't know what we are feeling, we feel 'bad' but we can't identify the feelings because they are so confused. A very high achieving pupil whose parents have high expectations of her may feel pleased that her friend has done really well in an exam but jealous because she didn't get top marks and then guilty because of her negative feelings and fearful of her parents' reaction. It is likely that she will want to hide the negative feelings but she can't stop them so they become bottled up. A child might be afraid that he will lose the love of his mother when she meets a new boyfriend and angry because he feels threatened by this new man, but these are difficult emotions to express clearly so they become muddled and that child's behaviour might change.

It is very important to consider the culture of the young people we work with. Emotions and expressions of emotions are subjective and dependent on the context of the speaker and listener and may reflect the sociocultural norms of both. It is important to understand a culture if we are to understand the emotions that are expressed by people of that culture (Bannerjee, 2005).

Being listened to and having the space to explore confused feelings with someone who isn't going to tell us to stop feeling angry or sad or afraid can help us to process our feelings and feel better about ourselves. It is so important, when talking to a child or young person about what they are going through, that we listen for the feelings, even when they are not labelled specifically. It is often the case that children don't know how they are feeling. They can't identify the bad feeling they have. It might be anger, fear or sadness but they will need someone who can recognise the feeling and help them to express and process it.

The most obvious way of acknowledging feelings is to ask the child or young person how they are actually feeling. Sometimes the young person will simply tell you and you can go on to explore that. Often, the young person might shrug their shoulders and say 'dunno'. They might say that they didn't care or they might give a very watered down version of their real feelings. They might say what they think you want to hear. In situations like these it is important not to tell the young person how you think they are feeling but it is possible to offer an idea of how they might be feeling tentatively. For example:

I'm wondering if you're feeling angry about what happened this morning?

It sounds like you're feeling sad about what happened with your dad.

I'm guessing it would have been pretty frightening when you heard your parents fighting.

The young person has to be given the opportunity to accept or reject those feelings. He might reply, 'No, I'm not sad, I'm more angry than sad' and so through the process of exploring those feelings you are enabling him to understand them more clearly. Rogers describes the way he checks his understanding with the client as 'catching just the colour and texture and flavour of the personal meaning you are experiencing right now' (Rogers, cited in Kirschenbaum and Henderson, 1989: 128).

Geldard and Geldard (2010) suggest that it is important not to over-use reflection of feelings as this is not a natural way of communicating for young people, who tend not to use reflection in their peer conversations. Prever (2011) suggests that reflection of feeling encourages the young person to consider their lives from a deeper perspective. In my experience, reflecting feelings is an important skill but it needs be used naturally, as a part of the normal flow of conversation.

Sometimes it can be easier for a young person to explore their feelings through drawing or music or role play. However they choose to communicate their feelings to you, the most important thing to do is to communicate your willingness to listen and to be there when they feel able to talk about what is going on for them.

Paraphrasing

Paraphrasing is the skill of rephrasing the important parts of what you have heard the young person say. It is a way of showing that you understand their point of view. In using this skill you will:

- Check your understanding of what they have said;
- Communicate the core qualities of acceptance and empathic understanding;
- Gain information about how they see themselves and their concerns;
- Build a trusting relationship (Culley and Bond, 2004).

You need to be accurate when paraphrasing and sometimes you might get it wrong so if you are not sure you can offer the paraphrase tentatively, using phrases like 'It sounds like …' or 'It seems that …' or 'I'm wondering if I've got that right'.

An example of paraphrasing would be:

Young person: I get so angry whenever I talk to my dad, it's like he doesn't listen to me at all. Then I go to school and my friends get on my nerves. I lose my temper, I take it out on them and they start to ignore me.

Helper: It sounds like it's hard to contain your anger and that ends up with you being ignored by your dad and your friends.

Summarising

Summaries are longer paraphrases and enable you to bring together the important aspects of what the young person has said in an organised way (Culley and Bond, 2004). Quite often a child or young person might want to talk about many things that are causing them distress. Life can seem overwhelming for all of us but particularly for a young person who is struggling with so many changes. They might talk in quite a chaotic way, jumping from one subject to another, digressing and changing their tone of voice. This can make it quite difficult to follow but it's often a reflection of the chaos in their lives and their swiftly changing moods. Summarising is useful when the conversation is coming to an end or when they've talked for quite a long time as it can help you and the young person to clarify what is going on for them. It can also serve to organise and prioritise what the problems and issues are. Here is an example of a summary that a helper uses after talking to a young person who is distressed about numerous relationships and problems at school:

So it sounds like your problems are overwhelming you. Your boyfriend has finished with you. Your friends are really unsupportive and seem to be siding with him. Your parents are arguing all the time and it feels like they don't have any time for you and on top of all that you have your GCSEs in a month and you don't know how to even start with revision. I'm wondering which of these feels like it's taking up the most space in your head at the moment?

Culley and Bond (2004) offer the following guidelines for paraphrasing and summarising:

- Be tentative and offer your perception of what the client has said.
- Avoid telling, informing or defining.

- Be respectful, do not judge, dismiss or use sarcasm.
- Use your own words; repeating verbatim may seem like mimicry.
- Listen to the depth of feeling expressed and match the level in your response.
- Do not add to what the client says, evaluate it or offer interpretations.
- Be congruent and don't pretend you understand.
- Be brief and direct.
- Keep your voice tone level. Paraphrasing in a shocked or disbelieving tone is unlikely to communicate either acceptance or empathy.

Questions

There are so many different kinds of questions which elicit so many different responses and it can be difficult to know what to ask and what impact the questioning might have on a young person who might be confused and distressed. More often than not it is enough to just listen without questioning. It is surprising how much one can learn by simply using reflection and paraphrasing. However, when working with children and young people it is inevitable that we will ask questions.

There are two main kinds of questions: open and closed (Geldard and Geldard, 2010):

Open questions: these are often questions which beginning with 'what', 'where', 'how' and 'who'. These are the most useful kinds of questions as they involve the young person more and encourage exploration and thoughtfulness. Try to avoid 'why' questions as they put pressure on the young person to justify his position.

Closed questions: these invite the young person to answer 'yes' or 'no', they are non-exploratory and tend to shut the conversation down.

In general it is better to use open questions but with children and young people who find it difficult to express themselves or who are shy or reluctant it is advisable to use closed questions at the beginning because they are much less threatening and complex and they can enable you to at least get a sense of what is going on for them. As they feel more comfortable it is likely that they will give fuller, more detailed answers.

Use of imagery

Sometimes young people are very good at talking about their feelings through imagery such as metaphor (Geldard and Geldard, 2010). A good example of this is when a girl might describe herself as feeling like she's on a roller coaster. This is a very common image but it can tell us a lot about those feelings and help that girl to understand her confusion of feelings if we stick with that image. It might help us to understand what happens during the up and down times. We could ask her to describe what it's like when she's climbing to the top; there might be dread, excitement, panic, fear. We could reflect on the idea that each time she goes down she knows it will be followed by a time of going up. We could talk about what it would be like if the ride were completely flat. Another really common image that people who are depressed use is the idea of feeling as if they are at the bottom of a dark pit. This can be a useful image to stay with because we can ask them to explore this feeling by asking what it feels like to be in that pit. We could start to explore ways out of the pit – are there footholds or vines or ropes? Working with an image in this way can demonstrate empathy with a young person's feelings and can really encourage them to look at their situation from a slightly different perspective.

Listening to silence

Silence can be awkward and threatening and uncomfortable but we can learn a lot from what young people do not say as well as from do what they do say (Culley and Bond, 2004). It is important to allow silences when we are talking to the children and young people who come to us asking for help. It is so natural in normal conversation to try to fill silences but in a therapeutic relationship it is essential to allow space for the young person or child to process their thoughts (Prever, 2011). It's possible that they will come to you obviously in distress but saying very little. When this happens it might well be enough for them to have a safe place to think, in the presence of someone who is trusted and undemanding. We can show that we are emotionally available to them by our non-verbal communication, our open and relaxed body language, our attentiveness through eye contact and the occasional encourager like a smile, a nod. It might be that they never open up but that they still seek you out – it's important to trust that they are benefiting from a relationship that allows them space to reflect without being pushed to speak about things that they are unwilling or unable to speak about.

Activity

Spend a week keeping a journal of the different interactions that you have had with friends, family, work colleagues and particularly any children or young people you come into contact with. Focus specifically on how well you have listened. Try to use some of the active listening skills that are suggested in this chapter and reflect on how they affected the interactions you had.

ACTIVE LISTENING WITH YOUNGER CHILDREN

When working with younger children it is important to keep in mind their developmental stage and to take into account the fact that their language and their understanding of language is usually not as mature as an older child's. Language should be kept simple and complex concepts and longer words should be avoided (McLeod, 2008). Workers should check out what they have understood as the child's meaning might be quite different from what the adult has understood. Body language is particularly important when working with younger children as they will pick up on situations when an adult's body language is at variance with the verbal message or the emotion expressed.

Play is central to a young child's world and learning to communicate through play is one of the most essential skills a worker can have. Watching a child at play, particularly fantasy play, can provide us with important insights into the child's inner world (Millar, 1968). However, it is unwise to start interpreting their play, particularly without appropriate training. It might be tempting to assume that a child who is repeatedly smacking a doll has been hit themselves but it might also be true that the child is enacting feelings of jealousy about a younger sibling. It is equally important to be alert to situations when a child's play seems to be communicating something inappropriate. Pithers (1990a: 20, cited in McMahon, 2009) states that 'Children cannot fantasize about events which lie completely outside of their experience'. This suggests that if a young child is acting out explicitly sexual behaviour it can be assumed that they have witnessed or even experienced it. There might be times when a child's behaviour causes concern and those responsible feel concerned that they might be communicating something worrying. If this is the case, it should not be ignored. It would be appropriate to speak to a line manager about your concerns and for them to consult with a child protection officer. Chapter 3 will give you more guidance on this.

Children love to play with adults, especially when the adults lose their inhibitions and play at the child's level. Children also enjoy having their solitary play witnessed by an adult (Meldrum, 2008). By entering into a child's fantasy world or by joining in their play we are communicating in an appropriate and effective way. Active listening skills like acknowledging and reflecting feelings are as important here as when listening to an older child. The following are some of the ways that we can use a child's normal play to help us to communicate with them:

- Playing house or doctors and nurses with a 3-year-old who then starts to pretend to cry in response to some imaginary event. We might say, 'Oh poor Lucy, you're really sad ... What made you feel sad?'
- Dressing up and role play can enable a child to re-enact experiences from their past or wishes for the future. This can then allow us to ask more about the child's experiences and encourage them to say more about them.
- Play with dolls or action figures can tell us about important relationships in that child's life and can enable us to communicate with the child in an age-appropriate and relevant way. Using symbols and figures to represent real people can help a child to explain a situation in a much less threatening way than direct questions. I will often ask a child to choose a figure to represent them and members of the family and to place them in a way that they see their family. It can also be used to show how they would like things to be. I will simply observe and reflect what I see.
- Scenes acted out by action figures can help us to model appropriate behaviour to a child who is displaying aggression to their peers. This is particularly effective if a favourite character from television is used. Peppa Pig is cross with George Pig and goes and talks to Mummy Pig instead of hitting George.
- Simple ball games help children to learn about turn-taking.

- Drawing and painting can help a child to express ideas and feelings that they might not have language for. Play doh is also very effective to help children to express feelings. I might ask a child to model some Play doh to show me what sad looks like or what angry looks like.
- A sand tray with symbols can be used very effectively to help children to create scenes and to change them. Patrick (2009: 17) describes a child playing with sand as an 'affirmation that the child can take control, has a sensitive and competent body and can make earth move'.

Allowing the child to take the lead in play, responding sensitively to their instructions and allowing ourselves to play at their level helps the young child to feel heard and encourages a sense of self-worth. McMahon (2009: 84) agrees that 'play is an important source of information about the child's inner world, and the child feels validated by our accepting and responsive response'.

BLOCKS AND BARRIERS TO EFFECTIVE COMMUNICATION

Sometimes it feels really difficult to establish a good rapport with the children and young people you work with or it might feel as if you have been listening but that you haven't really heard them. There are many ways in which good communication can be blocked and it is important to be aware of the blocks and barriers to good communication.

Activity

Think of times when you have found it really hard to listen to someone. What do you think are the blocks and barriers to therapeutic communication?

Some blocks might be external ones like:

- Tiredness
- Hunger
- Feeling ill
- Noise
- Inappropriate environment
- Young person's personal hygiene
- Client has learning disability or complex needs.

Other blocks are internal can sometimes be more difficult to deal with:

- Difference in culture and values
- Negative feelings towards the child or young person

- Other people's opinions about the young person
- Trying to hypothesise
- Working out what you're going to say next
- Getting upset about what the child or young person is saying
- Trying to find solutions
- Feelings of inadequacy
- Difficulties in your life
- Feeling unsafe.

These are just a few of the potential ways that can make listening and communicating effectively really difficult. With most of the physical and environmental blocks it is usually enough to be aware and responsive to them. Being congruent is important – pretending that you are feeling ok and not being able to listen well can be damaging to the relationship. Simply saying to a young person that you are finding it really hard to listen because of background noise and suggesting you go somewhere else or that you do a different activity is so much better than struggling on and risking them feeling that their concerns aren't being heard.

The psychological barriers are more complex and often we are not aware of how a relationship might be affected by internal blocks. This is where your own self-awareness is so important. It is essential to be aware of your own 'stuff' so that you can avoid responding to the client from your own frame of reference. Equally we should always try to be aware of the young person's frame of reference. Sometimes they might have views that are abhorrent to you. It is hard not to react to someone's prejudiced views but it's important to keep in mind that that young person was not born with those views; he or she learnt them from their environment. A young person's search for identity might lead them to align themselves with groups who hold extreme views. Remember that we can show empathy without having to agree with or like what the young person is saying.

There may be times when a young person is telling you things that upset you or cause you to worry about how to respond to them. They might well be asking you to sort their problems out for them. Perhaps you feel overwhelmed by what they are saying and feel you can't respond. In these situations you have to remember to use active listening skills. Your role is not to fix their problems, it is to listen and help them to find their own solutions.

When you do feel overwhelmed you need to recognise your limitations – it can be hard to carry around someone else's pain and anxiety. It can fill you up so you are no longer able to listen. It is essential to have support in your workplace to help you to process and deal with the emotional impact of working closely with young people who are experiencing emotional distress. 'Discussing your concerns with a colleague or line manager (within your confidentiality agreement) can be very helpful as they can offer you support, ease isolation and perhaps make suggestions that you have overlooked' (Donnelly and Neville, 2008: 68). Unfortunately in most Tier 1 settings there is not a formal supervision structure as there would be for a counsellor. Nevertheless, it is important that you do not try to take on too much and that you speak to a colleague regularly about how you are and how you are managing your relationships with the children and young people you are working with.

You also need to know when and how to refer on. If you recognise that a child or young person has specific mental health needs, you need to refer them to another person, agency or organisation that is better placed to offer support than yourself.

SELF-DISCLOSURE

The general guidelines when working therapeutically with people is not to disclose personal information about your life. In a relationship where your role is that of helper, your personal circumstances do not need to come into the relationship. If you have information or even feelings that you want to share with the young person, you should only do it if it is going to benefit the therapeutic relationship. For example, you might share your feelings of sadness about a situation a young person has told you about. It might be that they didn't say they were sad because they are trying to hide it but by sharing your feelings, you are encouraging the young person to explore their own sadness and maybe to realise that they are allowed to feel sad. If however you are sharing feelings that are not relevant to the young person's story, you are making the conversation about you, not them.

There is an argument however that suggests that when working with young people, a certain amount of self-disclosure is a good thing. Self-disclosure is a normal part of conversation and relationships are successful when people feel comfortable talking to others about their experiences, ideas and feelings. As an adult it is important to show the young person that you view them as an equal and that will mean talking about yourself and sharing feelings and experiences (Geldard and Geldard, 2010).

CONFIDENTIALITY AND DISCLOSURE

It can be really hard to gain the trust of a child or young person if they feel that you are going to tell someone else what they have told you. It's so important for us all to feel that if we tell something sensitive or private to someone, they will keep it to themselves. Trust has to be at the foundation of any good relationship and is an essential part of successful communication. The Ethical Framework for Good Practice in Counselling and Psychotherapy (British Association for Counselling and Psychotherapy, 2007) stresses the importance of confidentiality. The Nursing and Midwifery Council Code of Conduct states that: 'You must respect people's right to confidentiality' (2008).

It is also just as essential that as adults and professionals we ensure that the children and young people in our care are safe. We are duty bound to adhere to safeguarding policies and practices and to report any child protection issues such as abuse and neglect. When I first meet a young person I tell them that everything they tell me is confidential unless they tell me something which makes me feel that they or another child is not safe. I tell them that I will never go behind their back but that there are some things I can't keep to myself. I assure them that if that is the case, I will always tell them who I'm going to speak to. It might be that you risk that relationship but it is always more important to make sure that the child is safe from harm.

CONCLUSION

This chapter has shown that effective communication is vital if professionals are going to have meaningful, empathic, working relationships with the children, young people and families that they work with. Listening in a genuine, attentive and responsive way is a key part of therapeutic communication as is self-awareness and it is our responsibility as professionals to ensure that we show willingness to engage fully with those we come into contact with.

REFERENCES

Adler, R., Rosenfeld, L. and Proctor, R. (2007) *Interplay: The Process of Interpersonal Communication*. Oxford: Oxford University Press.

Argyle, M. (1988) *Bodily Communication*. London. Routledge.

Bannerjee, R. (2005) *Cultural Differences in the Experience and Expression of Emotion: Social and Emotional Aspects of Learning: Guidance*. London: DfES.

British Association for Counselling and Psychotherapy (2007) *Ethical Framework for Good Practice in Counselling and Psychotherapy*. Lutterworth: BACP.

Casemore, R. (2006) *Person Centred Counselling in a Nutshell*. London: Sage.

Culley, S. and Bond, T. (2004) *Integrative Counselling Skills in Action*. London: Sage.

Donnelly, E. and Neville, L. (2008) *Communication and Interpersonal Skills*. Exeter: Reflect Press.

Feltham, C. and Dryden, W. (1993) *Dictionary of Counselling*. London: Whirr Publishers.

Geldard, K. and Geldard, D. (2010) *Counselling Adolescents: The Proactive Approach for Young People*. London: Sage.

Gibbs, G. (1988) *Learning by Doing. A Guide to Teaching and Learning Methods. Oxford Centre for Staff and Learning Development*. London: Further Education Unit.

Hargie, O. (2011) *Skilled Interpersonal Communication: Research Theory and Practice*, 5th edn. London: Routledge.

Khuri, F. (2000) *The Body in Islamic Culture*. London: Saqi Books.

Kirschenbaum, H. and Henderson, V. (1989) (eds) *The Carl Rogers Reader*. London: Constable.

Koprowska, J. (2010) *Communication and Interpersonal Skills in Social Work*, 3rd edn. Exeter: Learning Matters.

McLeod, A. (2008) *Listening to Children: A Practitioner's Guide*. London: Jessica Kingsley.

McMahon, L. (2009) *The Handbook of Play Therapy and Therapeutic Play*, 2nd edn. London: Routledge.

Meldrum, B. (2008). Symbolic Play as a Medium of Change. *Counselling Children and Young People*. BACP, September: 24–9.

Millar, S. (1968) *The Psychology of Play*. Harmondsworth: Penguin.

National Autistic Society (2012) *What is Autism?* Available from: www.autism.org.uk (accessed 23 February 2012).

Nursing and Midwifery Council (2008) *The Code: Standards of Conduct, Performance and Ethics for Nurses and Midwives*. London: NMC.

Patrick, E. (2009) Sand Unlimited. *Counselling Children and Young People*. BACP, September: 17–22.

Prever, M. (2011) *Counselling and Supporting Children and Young People: A Person-centred Approach*. London: Sage.

Rogers, C. (1951) The Necessary and Sufficient Conditions for Therapeutic Change. *Journal of Consulting Psychology*, 21: 95–103.

Rogers, C. (1967) *On Becoming a Person: A Therapist's View of Psychotherapy*. London: Constable.

Rogers, C. (1986) Reflection of Feelings. *Person Centred Review*, 1 (4): 125–40.

Wood, J. (2004) *Communication Theories in Action: An Introduction* Belmont, CA: Wadsworth/Thomson Learning.

6

INTERVENTIONS WITH CHILDREN, YOUNG PEOPLE AND FAMILIES

ERICA PAVORD AND MADDIE BURTON

Overview

- Intervention models in CAMHS
- Identifying difficulties
- Therapeutic interventions
- Interpersonal psychotherapy and counselling
- The humanist approach including:
  - Person-centred approaches
- The psychodynamic approaches, including:
  - Parent–infant psychotherapy
  - Under-fives model
  - Play therapy
- The systemic approach including:
  - Systemic Family Therapy
- The behavioural approaches, including:
  - Cognitive behavioural therapy
- Psychopharmacology

(Continued)

(Continued)

With accompanying case studies including interventions for deliberate self harm, anorexia nervosa and depression.

INTRODUCTION

The chapter will focus on a sample of interventions typically used in CAMHS to support children, young people and families. The main theoretical models, psychodynamic, systemic, behavioural and humanistic, used in counselling and psychotherapy will be considered alongside some examples of recommended interventions. Interventions related to specific mental health presentations will be discussed with case studies. There are no specific activities in this chapter as readers are encouraged to read and reflect on the case studies provided.

It is very important to remember that essential to every intervention is the relationship between the young person and the individual supporting them. The relationship, and what emerges from it can be a 'potent dynamic' and is often more powerful in terms of bringing about change than the actual model of intervention adopted. The particular approach adopted will depend on a variety of factors relating to the individual and their context. What is different with CAMHS provision as opposed to adult mental health services is that in CAMHS, a *systemic* view is always adopted. The infant, child or young person is always considered in the context of their *system*, whatever the *system* the young person sits in; primarily their 'family' and their early years and school contexts. Thinking and working with all elements of the young person's system is crucial to understanding and bringing about positive change. In a similar way interventions within CAMHS are usually a combination of medical, psychological and systemic models. In adult mental health the primary model of intervention is medical. (In recent years there has been a slow move to a combined approach like the CAMHS model, with an increasing availability of psychological services, such as IAPT (Improving Access to Psychological Therapies), for adults and older adults.) It must be acknowledged that interventions can only be implemented by those qualified to do so who are also appropriately regulated and supervised by a professional body. That said, workers in all tiers should adopt a model of a collaborative, person-centred approach, one that is built on trust, respect and a non-judgemental position at all times.

CAMHS

The four-tier CAMHS model was discussed earlier. Child and adolescent mental health usually sits within a medical and psychological diagnostic model, therefore children and young people tend to receive a diagnosis if an assessment reveals this to be appropriate. This will be a primarily medical *interpretation* but the *approach* both to interpretation and treatment is one which considers all factors, both psychological and sociological. An appropriate treatment or intervention is then recommended according to the diagnosis. Freeth (2007, cited in Prever, 2011: 57) argues that this model does not sit well with the *person-centred* approach although CAMHS workers should be adopting a person-centred or *humanistic* approach where the focus is on relationship building alongside the treatment or intervention. Regardless of what sort of approach is used – cognitive behavioural therapy, eye movement desensitisation re-programming (which is receiving more attention for the treatment of post-traumatic stress disorder in CAMHS) or family therapy – the point is not to primarily pathologise an individual according to a diagnosis, but to adopt a person-centred relationship approach.

In 2008 CAMHS in the UK were reviewed and recommendations were given to improve their ability to meet the educational, health and social care needs of all children and young people at risk of, or experiencing, mental health problems. The review outlined the good practice and progress made since the introduction of the *National Service Framework for Children, Young People and Maternity Services* (Department of Health and Department for Education, 2004) and *Every Child Matters* (Department for Education and Skills, 2003). It also gave recommendations for how to improve services. It sought the opinions of children, young people and families who were involved with services and found that they are not always 'well known, accessible, responsive or child-centred'. They found that those who accessed specialist services did not always have 'the opportunity to develop trusting relationships with staff for the length of time they need'. There are variations in the service offered by different CAMHS teams across the country, some having unhelpful thresholds for referral criteria which can lead to inequalities in the level and type of service offered to children who have similar needs (CAMHS, 2008). It is clear that both universal (Tier 1), Tier 2 and specialist (Tiers 3–4) services for child and adolescent mental health need to engage with them effectively and provide flexible interventions which address their needs at an individual and developmentally appropriate level. Children, young people and their families need to know what is available, be listened to and be able to access help quickly and easily:

> What is clearly needed most is an interactive blend of therapies applied across the system that can foster optimum emotional and mental integration in children and adolescents. (Norton, 2011: 2)

The coalition government's document *No Health Without Mental Health* (HM Government, 2011) recommended that:

> ... care and support, wherever it takes place, should offer access to timely, evidence-based interventions and approaches that give people the greatest choice and control over their own lives, in the least restrictive environment, and should ensure that people's human rights are protected. (2011: 6)

In relation to the mental health needs of children and young people it stated that:

> Care and support should be appropriate for the age and developmental stage of children and young people, adults of all ages and all protected groups. (2011: 25)

It was universally acknowledged, as the CAMHS Review (2008) highlights, that accessing Tiers 3 and 4 can be problematic. This is in part now being addressed and extended to significant proportions of the country through the Children and Young People Improving Access to Psychological Therapies (CYP IAPT) project model which commenced in 2012. CYP IAPT works with existing CAMHS to:

- Improve access to CAMHS, and the partnership with children, young people, families, professionals and agencies;
- Build capability to deliver positive and measurable outcomes for children, young people and families;
- Increase choice of evidence-based treatments available.

It is a rolling model with service transformation at the heart with the voices of children and young people being instrumental in this process. Key is enhancement of the therapeutic relationship with children and families together with collaborative practice, this is seen as essential. Already 'self-referral' – the ability of a parent or child to refer themselves into CAMHS without needing a professional referral to access the service – has started. This is a really important element and includes an outreach service and partnership working with the education sector, which it is hoped will reach more children and young people needing help (CYP IAPT, 2012). It is anticipated that by 2013 over a third of under-19s will live in an area where CAMHS have been transformed. That is 4 million children and young people (Burstow, 2012). This represents a potential trend to start to reverse the statistics produced in 2004 when it was estimated 40% of children with a mental health disorder were not receiving any specialist service and that many more were experiencing problems but not having a diagnosis or access to specialist services (Department of Health and Department for Education, 2004). CYP IAPT had an initial focus on cognitive behavioural therapy (CBT) for anxiety disorders and parenting therapy for parents of 3- to 10-year-olds. The next programme includes evidence-based interpersonal psychotherapy and systemic family therapy for self-harm, eating disorders, depression and conduct disorders. Alongside current CAMHS changes are PbR (payment by results) proposals to bring CAMHS in line with adult and older adult PbR models which were introduced in 2012. These are powerful implications for CAMHS in that it is planned that clinical resources will only be available according to need and in relation to outcomes measures (PbR CAMHS, 2013; Royal College of Psychiatrists, 2012).

IDENTIFYING DIFFICULTIES

The people in the best position to recognise that a child or young person is experiencing mental health difficulties include the individual themselves, family members and workers in Tier 1 universal services – those who have contact on a regular basis: teachers, youth workers, health visitors, school nurses, GPs, social workers and so on. It is necessary for these professionals to have knowledge and understanding of child and adolescent mental health issues and the skills to identify signs of mental health problems and to know how to support and refer on to a service which is best placed to provide assessment and appropriate interventions.

School-based counselling (Tier 1) is an available and accessible form of psychological therapy for young people in the UK, with approximately 70,000–90,000 young people accessing services per year (British Association for Counselling and Psychotherapy, 2013). All secondary schools in Wales and most primary schools in Northern Ireland provide access to school-based counselling services. In fact, in Wales there is now a statutory duty for authorities to provide access to school-based counselling services and many areas provide therapeutic play interventions in primary schools. This was in response to the suicide cluster of young people in Bridgend, South Wales which reached a peak during 2007–2009.

With regard to younger children and families, children's centres offer timely and supportive community-based interventions. As well as support they provide opportunities for early identification of potential problems. Some of these interventions are described in Chapter 4.

In some cases, the problems will be significant and a referral to a GP or paediatrician and CAMHS is the most appropriate action. A GP is usually the first point of referral. Although, as we are now beginning to see, children and families will be able to self-refer to CAMHS. A GP can undertake a mental health assessment and then refer on as considered appropriate. For example, as a rough guide, a young person presenting with self-harming behaviour, suicidal ideation, deliberate self-harm, eating disorder, anxiety disorders, depression or psychotic behaviours would be referred to Tier 3. A young person presenting with behavioural difficulties or neuro-developmental problems would be seen in Tier 2 services. Often young people are initially seen in Tier 2 services and then referred on from Tier 2 to Tiers 3 or 4.

THERAPEUTIC INTERVENTIONS

Interventions in Tiers 2–4 usually include: family work, family therapy, parent work, parent groups, individual work and often a combination model of a psychological and pharmacological intervention and approaches.

Before going through the different approaches and models of therapeutic interventions, it is important to acknowledge that counselling and psychotherapy for children and young people is very different from the traditional adult approaches and needs to be developmentally appropriate, individualised, flexible and creative. It needs to engage young people who are often reluctant to talk or find it difficult to recognise or understand their feelings. The young person's context or system also requires attention as they are interrelated and one cannot function in isolation of the other. Typically a young person may be receiving support individually but ideally and if possible, this would also be alongside parent and family work.

Examples of creative, expressive and informal interventions for children and young people in use in all tiers include:

- Art therapy
- Drama therapy
- Adventure-based or wilderness therapy
- Narrative therapy
- Animal-assisted therapy
- Parenting interventions
- Mentoring.

INTERPERSONAL PSYCHOTHERAPY AND COUNSELLING

The main four theoretical models of counselling and psychotherapy are: *humanistic, psychodynamic, systemic and behavioural*. Increasingly counsellors and therapists are undertaking an integrative training which is a model integrating complementary aspects of all four models and is probably the most useful way forward in terms of developing an approach which addresses the needs of the individual. Individual therapeutic work with children and young people rarely involves a sole intervention and is usually alongside parent and family work. It is always about the appropriate application of a particular model to the young person and *not* the other way round: fitting the young person to the model.

HUMANISTIC APPROACH

The person-centred approach is the most widely known of the humanistic approaches, developed by Carl Rogers in the 1950s. This approach is covered to some extent in Chapter 5. Rogers' core conditions of empathy, unconditional positive regard and congruence tend to underpin all approaches of therapy and are the mainstay of the therapeutic relationship and effective communication. This section will deal with the theory behind the approach and look at how it is applied in work with a young person using a case study. The person-centred approach emphasises the therapeutic nature of human understanding so the self of the therapist and their deep acceptance of and respect for the child or young person as an individual is paramount (Prever, 2010).

The therapist working with a child or young person using the person-centred approach must provide a particularly special kind of relationship if he or she is to help that client to change and grow. Rogers identified six conditions which he felt were 'necessary and sufficient' for therapeutic growth. He believed that if these conditions were present in the relationship, they alone would bring about this change.

The six conditions are:

1. Two people are in psychological contact.
2. The first person, the client is in a state of incongruence, being vulnerable or anxious.
3. The second person, the therapist, is congruent or integrated in the relationship.
4. The therapist demonstrates unconditional positive regard for the client.
5. The therapist demonstrates an empathic understanding of the client's internal frame of reference and endeavours to communicate this to the client.
6. The communication to the client of the therapist's empathic understanding and unconditional positive regard is to a minimal degree achieved (Rogers, 1957).

Through the therapeutic relationship and the experience of the six conditions, the person-centred approach enables the child to become 'more resilient, more fulfilled more confident and more inclined to be all that they possibly can be' (Prever, 2011: 22).

It seems quite straightforward as the person-centred approach does not recommend a certain set of techniques and skills that have to be applied. It is the self of the therapist and the quality of the relationship that provide the experience of the six conditions. Existential psychotherapist Irving Yalom (1980: 5) notes that: 'It is the relationship that heals – it is the single most important lesson the therapist must learn.'

Chapter 5 summarises the main active listening skills that convey the quality needed in a person-centred therapist. Skills of reflection, paraphrasing and immediacy and the importance of positive body language all convey an empathic, warm, accepting and genuine attitude and help to build trust. The therapist's ability to sit with the client in their pain, fear or anger without trying to change it is key to building a therapeutic relationship that can, in time, facilitate change. The following case study illustrates how the relationship and the therapist's way of being is what enables the young person to gain a more robust sense of self.

Case study

Katie was a 17-year-old girl who had been in and out of care since she was 6 years old. She was angry with social workers, with her mum, with the school she had left the year before and with most of the well-meaning professionals that had tried to help her. Her housing support worker referred her to a counselling service because she had recently been given a flat of her own but found it impossible to move in there because she felt paranoid and anxious all the time. She was staying at her mum's house but their relationship was strained and she was feeling depressed. She couldn't go out at all unless she had drunk alcohol or taken amphetamines and when she did go out she would get into fights and end up feeling more angry, anxious and depressed. When she first started counselling she was very open with the details of her life but found it very difficult to talk about her feelings other than her anger, not because she didn't want to, more because she found it difficult to know

(Continued)

(Continued)

how she felt about her difficult experiences. For the first 8 to 10 sessions the thera-pist listened to Katie's story with empathic understanding, gently reflecting back Katie's memories and wondering what it had been like for her. The therapist didn't challenge Katie's anger towards everyone, she simply reflected Katie's feelings in an empathic way. Gradually, as Katie listened to her own story reflected back to her by the therapist she began to allow herself to feel emotions other than anger. When Katie spoke of her stepfather shouting and hitting her sister the therapist reflected how scary it would have made her if she'd been there, and Katie was able to acknowledge her fear. When Katie spoke of her feelings of protectiveness of her mother and sister, the therapist's reflections helped Katie to realise how strong and brave she'd been. Slowly, Katie's self-awareness and esteem began to emerge. She found it difficult to see this herself but she was able to start going out by herself more. Eight months after therapy started she passed her driving test and got a job. During this time Katie had started to trust the therapist and would allow herself to cry and feel that her sadness was justified. Towards the end of the therapy she reflected that she felt calmer and stronger because she knew that someone really believed in her.

THE PSYCHODYNAMIC APPROACHES

The psychodynamic approach has its roots in the work of Sigmund Freud (1856–1939), though there have been many other important figures who have taken his ideas into different directions. At the core of any psychodynamic approach is an interest in the unconscious processes of the mind. Therapists working in a psycho-dynamic way are concerned with the inner world which is made up of feelings, memories, beliefs and fantasies. Analysts working with children at the outset of the 20th century found that they were unable to describe their anxieties verbally and seemed not the least bit interested in exploring their past or accessing their uncon-scious minds through free association and dream analysis. Melanie Klein and Anna Freud, two major figures in the psychoanalytical world working with children, agreed that play was the medium through which children express themselves most freely (Landreth, 2002).

Child psychotherapy assesses and addresses the impact of the child or young per-son's internal reality or world on their external world through close observation of play and through relationships in the therapy room. Verbal language is not a prere-quisite. Much importance is placed on the therapeutic relationship and particularly on the feelings that are present in the way that the child relates to the therapist. These are called transference feelings and could be described as the unconscious feel-ings from important relationships in the child's life that are reflected in the way the child relates to the therapist. The therapist is able to make use of these feelings by trying to create an environment in which the child might experiment with new ways of relating (Hopper, 2006).

Child psychotherapy is a specialised Tier 3 service and can be long-term and quite intensive. Children may be seen for one to three 50-minute sessions per week over a variable period of time. There are short-term interventions such as the under-fives model described below. However, for some children and young people with complex mental health problems, long-term psychotherapy may be the preferred and appropriate option.

Parent–infant psychotherapy

The current coalition government has emphasised the need for services to intervene as early as possible to avoid future mental health problems, and so it seems obvious that interventions offered to mothers and their babies who are experiencing problems are essential if baby is to develop in an emotional healthy way (Allen, 2011). The mental health of under-fives and their parents and early intervention have become increasingly under the spotlight over the past 20 years (Pozzi-Monzo et al., 2011). Chapter 4 outlined some of the Tier 1 interventions that aim to promote and prevent mental health problems in babies and young children, but unfortunately there are times when the issues are deep set and a more targeted and intensive intervention is needed to try to repair the attachment relationship between mother and baby.

Parent–infant psychotherapy sits in Tier 3 although service provision is by no means widespread and is only available in some parts of the country. It was pioneered by Selma Fraiberg (1980). The theoretical foundations are in Freudian psychoanalysis and it is concerned with the mind's unconscious processes. In this approach, the patient is the relationship between a parent and baby rather than an individual. Through therapy the parent gains insight and understanding which facilitates change and helps her become more attuned to her baby's needs. The idea is that if parents are able to understand and make sense of their difficult early experiences, they are less likely to replicate those experiences in their child's life. A core component of this approach is the therapist's effort to understand how the mother's current and past experiences impact on her feelings and behaviour towards her baby. Fraiberg describes the mother's past, often traumatic experiences as 'ghosts in the nursery', which play out in her relationship with her baby so that she is unable to attend to the baby's emotional needs without confusing them with her own childhood needs. To illustrate these ideas it is useful to imagine a mother who is suffering from the effects of the trauma of domestic violence. On hearing the hungry cries of her baby she perceives them as angry outbursts of aggression (mirroring her abusive partner) and responds with fear or anger, frightening her baby. Through the gentle explorations of these feelings with the therapist, the mother is able to separate her own feelings from those she projects onto her baby and she begins to understand and respond appropriately to the baby's cries.

Case study

The following case study is taken from a paper written by parent–infant psycho-therapist Amanda Jones (2006). It has adapted and simplified a very complex case in order to illustrate the main processes that take place in parent–infant psychotherapy.

Farida was referred to a parent–infant psychotherapist by adult mental health and social services. She had been receiving therapy for depression and post-traumatic stress disorder following a very violent incident with her baby's father when she was pregnant. He was sent to prison following the incident but Farida had been depressed ever since and after the birth of her baby boy, Amani, she had been experiencing frightening flashbacks, disturbed sleep, explosions of anger and periods of dissociation. Her relationship with her baby was extremely fragile. She had the support of her mother and it was because of this that she was able to keep the baby who was on the Child in Need Register. Following a course of cognitive behavioural therapy for her PTSD, the symptoms decreased but Farida was still depressed and very anxious because she felt that she was unable to bond with her 8-month-old baby. Amani cried frequently and seemed to reject Farida's attempts to comfort him. He would sometimes lash out at her either with his arms or by banging his head against hers. In response, she would thrust him away from her, putting him down and withdrawing her attention. He would increase his crying until he fell into exhausted sleep. She went through the motions of caring for him, providing for his immediate needs, feeding and changing him but there was little to no eye contact and even when she tried to comfort him by rocking and patting, she gave no indication through verbal or non-verbal communication that she was in tune with his needs. In observing both conscious and unconscious behaviours, the therapist finds a way of helping Farida to make sense of her experience and how her responses to Amani affect him. This is done in a gentle, sensitive way so that Farida doesn't feel blamed or responsible, she is simply able to see what her baby might be communicat-ing with his behaviour and why. Through her interventions the therapist gives voice to Amani's distress and gives a context for Farida's response to him. As the therapist listens empathically to Farida talking about her traumatic relationship she also ensures that Farida is noticing what Amani is doing and reminds her of the reality of him as a baby rather than as a representation of his violent father. The therapist remains alert to any signs of positive interaction between Farida and Amani and shows Farida the impact it has on Amani's way of relating to her. Moments when she responds to his attempts to engage her like a quick game of peek-a-boo give Farida a window of possibility about how she could relate to him differently. A quick kiss planted on his head is focused on and the therapist reflected how it seemed that Farida is more able to relate to him like the little baby he is. During the moments when Amani communicated his distress, the therapist was able to comfort him by stroking him and reassuring him that his mother was there and soon Farida was able to do the same.

(Adapted and simplified from Jones, 2006)

Under-fives model

The 'Under-Fives Service' is a brief psychoanalytical model based on a service first developed in the Child and Family Department of the Tavistock Clinic in the late 1970s. It offers up to five sessions to families where there are concerns and anxieties over a baby or child under five. It is considered a specialist service and sits in Tier 3 CAMHS. Clinicians working in the model would include child psychotherapists and others such as psychologists and nurses. Reasons for referral typically include: temper tantrums and aggression, soiling and sleeping problems and behavioural problems in Early Years settings. As parents tell their story they are often able to make links between the experiences they and the child had together. The children give clear demonstrations of their own struggle through their play (a specific set of toys is used for all families) and thinking about this helps parents understand their child. By observing and sharing observations with parents thinking is facilitated (Miller, 2008). Some problems may seem minor but if taken seriously with an effort to understand what is being communicated, parents can feel more able to cope and the child less anxious, and subsequently behaviours will often subside, thus avoiding escalation on the part of the child and diminished parenting capacity. The process of thinking together and endeavouring to make sense of what is happening supports parents, enabling children to feel more contained with a shift in patterns of relating that have previously been unhelpful.

Play therapy

The Association for Play Therapy (2013) has defined play therapy as:

> ... the systematic use of a theoretical model to establish an interpersonal process wherein trained play therapists use the therapeutic powers of play to help clients prevent or resolve psychosocial difficulties and achieve optimal growth and development.

Play therapy seeks to provide a troubled child space where he or she can feel safe enough to explore feelings and thoughts through play in the presence of a therapist who creates a safe and accepting atmosphere through empathically listening. Above all the therapist must show patience, respect and honesty and give the child an experience of having their viewpoints and experiences sensitively listened to and understood. As with all therapeutic approaches, the therapeutic relationship is the key to facilitating change.

Critical to successful play therapy is the playroom and materials. The playroom should have an atmosphere of warmth and acceptance and convey a clear message: 'This place is for children. You are free to use what is here. Be yourself. Explore' (Landreth, 2002).

Children will usually find a playful use for just about anything but a well-stocked playroom helps. Items such as:

- Dolls houses with figures
- Drawing, painting and arts and crafts
- Sand trays
- Puppets
- Mini figures, toys, animals, vehicles, fences, trees, shells, stones, feathers, pretend food.

Landreth (2002) explains that toys should be selected that promote clear understanding for the therapist and allow the child to represent themes of real life, aggression and creative expression which will help clear communication between child and therapist.

During the therapeutic session the child is free to choose to play with whatever they wish to play with and the therapist observes the child in an active and involved way. Landreth (2012) demonstrates via a DVD an example of child-centred play therapy which is useful to watch. The therapist does not have to make sense of the play as much as feeling and emotionally connecting with what it is like to be in the child's place. Inevitably the therapist will be drawn into interpreting the child's play but it is important to remember that the child alone is the authority on what is happening. If an interpretation is shared with the child and is completely wrong, the child would be led away from their internal world and into the world of the therapist (Hopper, 2006). When the child represents their inner world and significant people with symbols and objects there is a sense of safety. If the therapist suggests that they know what or who the symbol is representing, that thing or person becomes reality and therefore unsafe: 'The therapist will not reach the hidden meanings unless she can stay with the child's symbols' (Hopper, 2006: 62).

Case study

Pippa was an 8-year-old girl referred to CAMHS by an educational psychologist. Pippa was an elective mute. She had been living in care for a year after living in a home where she had experienced neglect and abuse. She was hostile and aggressive towards everyone who came into contact with her, preferring to stay in her bedroom or in the corner of the classroom by herself. She was referred for play therapy as a way of helping her to express her feelings in a non-verbal way. For three months she came to weekly sessions and chose to play with a variety of toys and materials. The therapist observed her as she chose a toy and took herself off to a corner of the room to play without the therapist being able to see what she was doing. During the fourth and fifth month she seemed to choose the puppets more and more. She started to move around the room putting them in various different places and then going back to them, smiling and nodding to them. Although there was no verbal interaction Pippa had begun to show an interest in having some interaction. Gradually, Pippa started to approach the therapist with the puppets and the therapist would pretend to listen to them. The third time this happened the therapist quietly told Pippa that the puppet had said that it liked to see her smile and wanted her to know that it wanted to play with her. Pippa began to whisper very quietly to the puppets, making sure that the therapist couldn't hear. Soon it was clear from Pippa's face that the puppets had started to whisper back to her and the therapist tentatively wondered what they were saying. Pippa began to tell the therapist what the puppets were telling her. She said that they knew the bad things that had happened to her and that they wanted to tell the therapist. Bit by bit, Pippa, through the puppets, told the therapist about the physical and sexual abuse that she had experienced. She explained that she wanted to make friends with other people but was frightened to trust them in case they betrayed her. Gradually Pippa was able to explore her traumatising experiences and start to try out what it might be like to interact with other people in a positive way. The therapy was a way for Pippa to rehearse what it might be like to talk to real people in the world outside the playroom.

(Adapted from Hopper, 2006: 86)

It is important to acknowledge that this sort of work would only take place once a young person was living in a supportive, containing and understanding environment and parallel work with parents or carers would also take place. Not only does the therapeutic environment have to be containing and robust, so does the home environment. Therapy 'stirs things up' and can evoke strong emotions; environments outside the 'therapy room' need to be able to safely contain the child.

The systemic approach

The systemic approach incorporating family therapy is used most often in CAMHS settings. It focuses not on the intra-personal processes of an individual but on the interpersonal processes within the family. This approach sees the child or young person as part of a wider system, usually the family, and emphasises family relationships as an important part of psychological health.

The basic assumption underpinning all versions of family therapy is that the distress or maladjusted behaviour of individual family members is best understood as a manifestation of something going wrong at a systemic level: for example through ineffective communication between family members or some distortion of the structure of the family group. (McLeod, 2003: 191)

Three main schools of family therapy emerged out of this early systems thinking:

- Minuchin's structural family therapy
- Haley's strategic family therapy
- The Milan school of family therapy.

The Milan approach is most similar to the approaches found in current CAMHS settings although post-Milan there have been other influences which have become integrated into the way that family therapy is practised today.

Traditionally systemic family therapy is carried out by a team of therapists and aims to help bring about change by highlighting the role of the family or other members of the client's system in problem resolution (Hedges, 2005). Therapists must seek to maintain neutrality, which is not always an easy task. The classic format is for one or two therapists to sit with the family in a room with a two-way mirror, behind which sit the reflecting team of therapists. The reflecting team can interrupt the therapy through the use of a phone to offer reflections, ideas and suggestions to the lead therapist and the family. The team approach ensures that multiple perspectives are heard and considered. Children and young people can also take part in this, not only in the therapy room but also observing with the reflecting team, which can feel quite playful at times and empowering for them.

Genograms

Genograms are often a feature of family therapy and are a very helpful tool to use to gather information at an initial meeting and thereafter to keep in mind. They can be used beyond 'family therapy' as a way of history taking and understanding family systems. Children and young people enjoy the focus and involvement of the visual effect of drawing their family tree on a large sheet of paper, rather than answering questions. Genograms are able to consider family members and relationships both in the room and not in the room. Family systems can be very complex. Generational themes are often revealed and it means that problems can be seen and may be occurring, as part of the bigger picture or *system* (Burnham, 1986). Genograms can also be used to think about the other professionals and agencies involved with the family. Detail should include:

- Names and ages of family members
- Notable significant events including: dates of birth, marriages, separations and deaths
- Occupations
- Three generations – the young person, siblings, their parents and both sets of grandparents
- Children and young people like to also include any pets or other significant friendships.

Figure 6.1 shows the genogram for 'John's' family. You will see he has two older sisters and both maternal and paternal grandparents. There is an uncle on the maternal side who is separated from John's aunt as the transverse line indicates.

The systemic approach is guided by the idea that families become entrenched in certain ways of functioning and behaving which are more or less helpful to different members of the family. The aim of the therapy is to introduce new ideas and perspectives that will help family members to see familiar problems from new

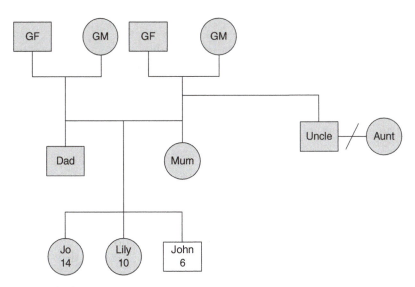

Figure 6.1 John's genogram

positions. Family therapy helps families to free themselves from a blaming culture where one family member is seen as the instigator of the problems. The Milan approach developed the therapeutic stance of *curiosity*, the assessment technique of *hypothesising* and the interviewing technique of *circular questioning* which has become so influential in family therapy and which ensures that multiple perspectives are heard and considered (Prevatt, 1999).

Curiosity

When the therapists working with the family are curious, they remain open to multiple ideas about what might be going on. It is natural when working with problems for us to look for solutions. Curiosity encourages the therapists and family to remain curious about what is happening because when we assume we have an explanation which might be useful for one member of the family, we give up looking for other descriptions which might be more useful for another member of a family (Cecchin, 1987). For example, a family might seek the help of CAMHS and want an explanation for their son's difficult and unpredictable behaviour. He is given a tentative diagnosis of ADHD which makes them feel better because they have an explanation for his behaviour, but in practice nothing changes, the family are still exhausted and the child is now labelled and unhappier than he was before. This single diagnosis has closed down the potential for other explanations and ideas about how to alleviate this family's difficult situation.

Hypothesising

A way of ensuring that therapists remain neutral and curious is to formulate hypotheses based on the information they have gathered about the family (Palazzoli et al., 1980). The initial hypothesis gives the therapist a starting point with the family and a focus for the questions. The hypothesis serves to further understanding and to introduce potential new meaning to the family. It does not have to be true, the therapists might have multiple and contradictory ideas (Jones, 1993):

> The value of a hypothesis is not in its truth but in its ability to create a resonance with those involved. (Cecchin, 1992: 90)

Shifting the perspective of the family about an issue that causes conflict can become an agent for change. Throughout the therapy, the hypotheses will change as more information becomes available and they remain useful in that they open up ideas and give the family alternative views of what might be happening.

Circularity

In order to test out a hypothesis the therapist uses circular questioning to explore this hypothesis with the family. Circular questions 'seek to connect what one family member does, thinks or wants with another family member' (Rivett and Street, 2009: 142). In a family where a child is having a lot of unpredictable, tearful tantrums the therapists might have a hypothesis that anger is not tolerated but sadness is listened to. These might include questions similar to the following:

> To Dad: 'How do the members of this family show that they are sad or angry?'
>
> To oldest daughter: 'If I were to ask Mum who is most sad in this family, what do you think she would say?'
>
> To youngest daughter: 'Who notices that you are sad first?'
>
> To Mum: 'What does your husband do when your daughter is sad?'

These circular questions help to elicit more information about how the family respond to sadness. They encourage each member to see and think about the issue from an alternative perspective and help the family members see that they all have different experiences or ideas about the tantrums.

The Milan school proposed that circular questioning in itself was therapeutic and could bring about change. Through careful questioning, based on hypotheses, the family members are able to recognise the patterns of behaviour and responses that they have been stuck in and gradually make changes which help them to create alternative ways of being (Palazzoli et al., 1980).

BEHAVIOURAL APPROACHES

Cognitive behavioural therapy

One of the most widely used approaches in mental health settings with both adults and children is cognitive behavioural therapy (CBT). CBT has two main influences, behaviour therapy and cognitive therapy. CBT with children and young people combines both components (Fuggle et al., 2013). There is a wealth of evidence-based research suggesting that CBT is an effective way of helping people to understand and manage unhelpful behaviours (Bonham, 2004). NICE guidelines recommend 'talking therapies' such as CBT as treatment for:

- Eating disorders (NICE, 2004a)
- Psychosis (bipolar disorder) (NICE, 2006)
- Depression (NICE, 2005)
- Social anxiety disorders (NICE, 2013)
- ADHD (NICE, 2008).

CBT is often recommended in these cases because it has the most robust scientific evidence across many psychological disorders. However, it is interesting to note young people have said in the Chief Medical Officers Report (DH, 2013: 100) that CBT, now usually offered as standard, does not work for everyone. A person-centred approach would be mindful of this when choosing an intervention in collaboration with the young person. Other therapies such as systemic family therapy are also recommended (Sanders and Wills, 2005).

CBT is an approach based on the idea that how we feel and what we do is in response to the way we think. CBT therapists will encourage children and young people to become more aware of how their thinking affects their feelings and behaviour and show them how to identify unhelpful, irrational and distorted thoughts and replace them with more flexible, accurate and evidence-based ones (Neenan and Dryden, 2006). It is a collaborative approach to therapy where the child or young person and therapist work together and the child or young person takes an active role in identifying and testing the validity of the thoughts which are causing them to behave in particular way. CBT sessions last for about 30–60 minutes each (Fuggle et al., 2013). The goals of therapy are arrived at after discussion between the therapist and young person and the focus of the therapy is the problem as the young person sees it rather than how other people experience it, which is an important point. Once the problem and goal have been identified, the therapist and the young person work together to challenge the negative thoughts maintaining the problem.

The CBT model (Beck, 1976):

- Highlights the role of cognitions (the process of knowing, learning and remembering) in determining emotions and behaviour.
- Cognitions may be dysfunctional, maladaptive or distorted.
- Altering or restructuring cognitive processes should lead to changes in emotions and behaviour.

Key principles

Core beliefs are developed in childhood and involve rigid ideas about the self, others and the world. For example: 'I'm worthless', 'I'm a failure', 'The world is a dangerous place'.

Cognitive assumptions form the basis for how we judge our world and how we predict what will happen. For example: 'No one likes me so I will be left out.' 'If ... then ...' statements are often used to make predictions based on our beliefs: *'If* I let myself get close to someone, *then* I will get hurt.'

Negative automatic thoughts (NATs) are automatic and largely unchallenged thoughts that enter the conscious mind. They are invariably negative: unhelpful, preoccupying and distorted and prevent us from doing what we want or need to do.

Cognitive formulation

An important part of the therapeutic work involves the problem formulation which therapist and young person create together. Fuggle et al. (2013) suggest that the assessment should only collect the information needed to understand the problem enough to plan an intervention; it is not always necessary to undertake extensive assessments. For many it is enough to come up with a maintenance formulation (see below) which provides sufficient information to gain understanding and to start the process of experimentation and change. For some, a deeper understanding of how the problems came about will be needed and a case formulation or onset formulation which includes important early experiences will help to give a context for the problems (Stallard, 2009). This helps the young person to understand the context of their problem; their early experiences that have impacted on their beliefs and the assumptions they make about the world and their relationships. They then see how certain trigger events will activate the beliefs and then lead to the maintenance of the problem. The maintenance and case formulation is shown in the case study below.

Case study

Leon was a 14-year-old boy who struggled with a number of issues. He was having problems in school, he found it difficult to concentrate and his teachers were concerned. He had started to find it irritating to be around friends as he would lose his temper and they would wind him up. He had stopped meeting up with them outside school. His mother had noticed that he was more withdrawn at home, he wasn't eating much and had started checking windows and doors at night and found it difficult to get to sleep as he was worried that lights had been left on. He agreed to go and see the school counsellor and together they talked about what Leon thought the problem was. He was fed up with feeling low, he found his friends annoying and he worried about how safe his mum was at home because his dad had only recently left and was living with another woman. Together, Leon and the therapist came up with the goals of getting on better with his friends and feeling more relaxed at home. They started with a maintenance formulation (Figure 6.2). Leon started to understand how his thoughts impacted on his feelings, both physi-

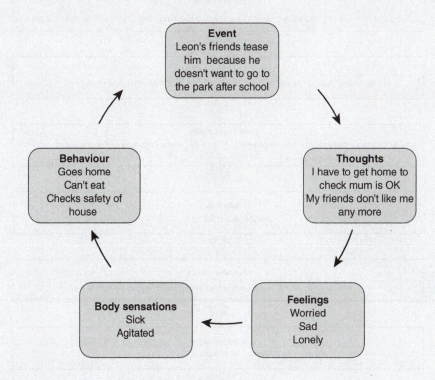

Figure 6.2 Leon's maintenance formulation

cal and emotional. In turn he saw how this impacted on his behaviour leading to him feeling more isolated and low in mood. He was frustrated with this because he didn't know why he felt his mum couldn't be safe in the house. The therapist talked to him more about his experiences at home and found out about his parents' marriage break-up. This enabled her to work with Leon to create a case formulation which helped him to understand the background to his feelings. The formulation is changeable and dynamic and can be adapted when new information is shared but it provides a rationale for Leon which the therapist can use to help him to challenge his unhelpful cognitions (see Figure 6.3).

The therapist started to work with Leon on some of the negative and unhelpful thoughts he had. She helped him to identify thinking errors, challenge thoughts, collect evidence for certain thoughts, and consider alternative, more helpful

(Continued)

(Continued)

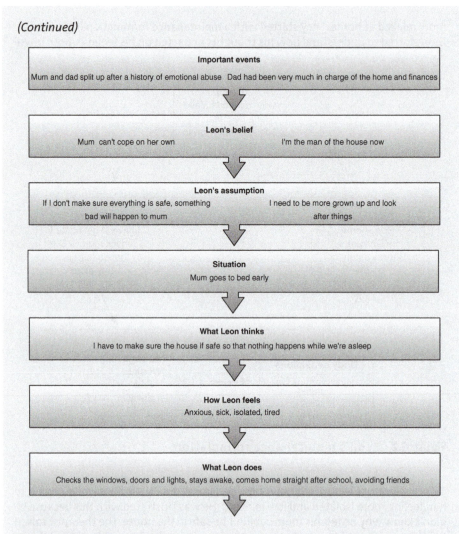

Figure 6.3 Leon's case formulation

(Adapted from Stallard, 2009)

thoughts (Stallard, 2002). When Leon began to really question the idea that his thoughts were facts, the therapist tried a behaviour experiment with him. They decided that when his friends asked him to go to the park, he would go. They talked through his expectations of what might happen to mum and thought about how he would feel when he went to the park. He decided that he was 70% certain that his mum wouldn't cope on her own and 50% certain that his friends would get on his nerves and he'd want to leave. They agreed that he would go for one hour and that mum would text him once to reassure him that everything was fine. After the experiment he reported that he had felt very anxious but he had managed to stay in the park and had enjoyed being with his friends. He decided that he now felt about 50% certain that his mum couldn't cope and only about 20% certain that his friends would get on his nerves. They continued to work together to challenge some of his thoughts about being safe at home.

As already stated a CAMHS model is always about the child in context, as part of a wider system. Children and young people are usually one part of a wider family and are often relatively powerless to change their situation unless their family are supportive of the changes. Looking back to the case study describing Leon's work with the CBT therapist, we can see that it would have been hard for him to maintain his confidence if his mother had been very anxious herself and undermined all his attempts to make changes. A systemic approach would see Leon and his mother and father, if possible together and focus on the family functioning rather than on Leon's intra-personal processes. Often families can be a maintaining factor and inadvertently collude with the young person's presentation so it is good practice to carry out individual work alongside parents and family members if appropriate.

PSYCHOPHARMACOLOGICAL INTERVENTIONS

Psychopharmacology includes drugs which influence psychological and mental states. They bring about changes in: mood, sensation, thinking, behaviour and the alleviation of symptoms, particularly in the treatment of mental disorders (psychiatric medication). Psychopharmacological interventions are a medical model of treatment and would be used in CAMHS settings together with a 'talking' therapy or psychological intervention. For mild, moderate or severe depression the first line treatment is a psychological therapy of at least three months' duration with guidance that medication is only to be offered in combination with a psychological therapy (NICE, 2005). Typically the most frequent medications prescribed in CAMHS are methylphenidate for ADHD, SSRIs (selective serotonin re-uptake inhibitors) for depression, anxiolytics for the management of anxiety and anti-psychotics (Dogra et al., 2009). Anti-psychotics are sometimes prescribed for the management of aggressive behaviour and conduct disorder (Loy et al., 2012).

INTERVENTIONS WITH YOUNG PEOPLE WHO DELIBERATELY SELF-HARM

... long term relationships with workers rather than offers of time limited work provide continuity and the chance to build rapport. I want workers to be more concerned about me, genuinely, than only thinking about risks. (Mental Health Foundation, 2006: 69)

The above personal testimony was made by a young person and included in the *Truth Hurts* report of an inquiry into self-harm among young people. As mentioned previously there has been a tendency in the past to focus on risk alone rather than considering risk within the context of an act of self-harm. When a young person who self-harms is referred to CAMHS an accurate assessment and understanding of the young person's internal world are crucial and must be critical, in order to manage and treat such young people (Bell, 2000). Without a thorough psychosocial assessment, one cannot conclude upon what an intended outcome may have been. NICE (2004b) guidelines recommend this sort of assessment within 48 hours of admission to hospital, by a CAMHS clinician. The clinician would then make a decision about discharge in conjunction with both the young person and their family. Key considerations are intent and motivation, therefore it is important to ask questions such as: what did you think was going to happen? For how long and what sort of preparations have you been making? A response may be that the young person who has taken an overdose thought they would go to sleep and not wake up. Taking the overdose may have been an impulsive act in contrast to someone who has been collecting tablets over a period of time. The therapeutic relationship is established at the assessment and would continue following on as ongoing treatment in future work. As reflected by Campbell and Hale (1991), therapy starts immediately. In this way the therapist becomes a part of the original chaos and remains alive in the mind of the young person. Essentially assessment and treatment need to be inextricably linked (Berman and Jobes, 1991), although this is often not the case. CAMHS teams have rotas for assessing cases admitted to hospital and do not necessarily take the young person onto their case load but may well refer back to the CAMHS team and allocate the case to another clinician.

Understanding how the young person manages stress is crucial. Current presentations are typically symbolic of earlier childhood difficulties, whether or not these are thought about and described in terms of attachment or relationship problems. These presentations and behaviours are evidence of earlier experiences of interpersonal, familial and relationship difficulties leading to insecurity of attachment (Briggs, 2002). So it is not surprising that looked after children carry an increased risk of self-harming behaviours, as discussed in Chapter 1.

We need to understand this more fully if we are to genuinely help. This can only be achieved with a thorough assessment. What we are initially presented with and what is observed about the young person's relationships with parents and peers provide vital clues in building a picture. The immediate factors we see about the parent/young person/peer relationship contributes to our understanding (Wohl, 1995).

Interventions would include any or a selection from the models discussed earlier in the chapter. One important principle is that of containment and holding by the therapist no matter which model of intervention is adopted. It is worth remembering, however, that many young people never have access to specialist services and may be first noticed in Tier 1 settings, schools for example. In these cases, it is important to seek advice from CAMHS professionals. Very often CAMHS clinicians work jointly with staff such as school nurses and counsellors.

The following case demonstrates the complexity of working with young people and provides clues to some contributory factors to self-harming behaviour.

Case study

Hazel is now 18. She was initially referred to CAMHS following admission to the local paediatric ward following an overdose when she was 16. Exam stress had been the reason given for the trigger precipitating her overdose. Previous history included being sent to boarding school when she was 13, where she had been very unhappy, only staying for a year. During this time she was referred to CAMHS local to the boarding school, and was diagnosed with ADHD. Hazel did not present with ADHD symptoms at the time of her overdose, neither did she agree with her diagnosis. Hazel chose to continue with the prescribed medication (methylphenidate) until she finished her exams, acknowledging it helped with concentration.

Hazel and her mother had experienced a traumatic birth with mum being traumatised and then suffering further with postnatal depression for quite a time. Alongside ongoing individual work with Hazel, mum and Hazel were seen together on occasions. It felt these sessions facilitated mum being able to make some repairs with Hazel, and for Hazel being able to discuss her own experiences with her mother. Mum had felt guilty about her poor bonding experience with Hazel. Despite these poor beginnings for both of them mum did have a capacity for thinking which enabled a significant improvement. Hazel no longer self-harms nor has she attempted another overdose and is getting on with life. She has since been discharged.

INTERVENTIONS EXAMPLES FOR YOUNG PEOPLE WITH ANXIETY DISORDERS, DEPRESSION AND ANOREXIA NERVOSA

The following case study revisits Jean, who was diagnosed with school phobia and depression (see Chapter 1). The description of the interventions used with Jean demonstrates the systemic approach which pays attention to her family and school context. In therapeutic work one of the most powerful precursors of change is through parents and their changed behaviours. In Jean's case there were several CAMHS clinicians involved as well as the incontinence service in Tier 1.

Jean was prescribed an SSRI as a medical treatment and intervention for depression. The consultant child and adolescent psychiatrist would be managing that aspect of Jean's treatment. Alongside her medical treatment individual work was undertaken with Jean by another CAMHS clinician. The individual worker would also engage with the school setting in addressing what was required in order for Jean to feel safe to attend. Jean had a rational reason for not attending, given her

(Continued)

(Continued)

experiences of bullying there. A combination of a CBT and interpersonal psycho-therapy model was used. The CBT approach would work out the 'problem': Jean's ideas around being fearful of incontinence which led her to not want to leave the house. Interpersonal therapy provided ongoing support and containment. Another CAMHS clinician worked with the parents in a similar way, challenging ideas they had about being accepting of what was 'dealt out' in life.

Jean's case demonstrates a typical example of several CAMHS clinicians working with the young person and family and the wider context of school and other health professionals. Periodically Jean and her family and the involved clinicians would all meet together for a review. The following example of an intervention for a young person with anorexia nervosa shows how the whole family are involved with the treatment in a Tier 3 or 4 setting. The Maudsley Approach as shown below is a combination of a behavioural and a family systems approach. Alongside this intervention the young person would receive other talking therapies including inter-personal therapy, perhaps CBT and the whole family would also be offered and expected to take part in Family Therapy as per NICE (2004) guidelines.

THE MAUDSLEY APPROACH

NICE guidelines state that family interventions that address the eating disorder should be offered to children and adolescents with anorexia nervosa (NICE, 2004a). This would include both behavioural treatment approaches and family therapies. The following case study looks not at a particular case but at a specific model developed and practised at the Maudsley hospital in London and at specialist centres in the USA, Canada and Australia. The Maudsley Approach is not family therapy as such but is a *family-based treatment* of adolescent anorexia nervosa which integrates principles and skills from many of the major schools of family therapy and is suitable for adolescents where there is less than three years' duration of anorexia nervosa (Maudsley Parents, 2013). It is used in conjunction with re-feeding programmes in both Tiers 3 and 4 services.

The approach is separated into three phases:

Phase 1: Re-feeding the young person

The family is tasked with helping the child to gain weight and restore healthy eating practices. Modelling empathy and understanding, the therapist encourages the parents to take control of their child's food intake through empathic but firm instruction. Family meals are taken at the clinic and the therapist observes the family's typical interaction patterns around eating. Parents take charge of the mealtime and siblings are encouraged to align themselves more with their sister, showing their understanding of how hard it is for her. This is an important part of the work; using Minuchin's structural ideas, helping the family to form appropriate parental and sibling subsystems. This phase can last up to 12 or more weeks as the family adjust to their roles and ensures that the child is regaining weight and developing healthier eating patterns. The therapist takes note of family interactions that are unhelpful. Parent and sibling subsystems are reinforced and attention is paid to any attempts to criticise the child or to any strong emotion expressed about the child's eating. When parents criticise or get emotional with their child it is reframed or *externalised* as the anorexia taking control. They are reminded that the anorexia is the one to blame, not the child or the parents.

Phase 2: Negotiating for a new relationship

Once the young person has regained weight and accepts her parents' demands that she eat, the therapist encourages the parents to start to give back some of the control over eating to their daughter. The therapist still supports the parents in their attempts to feed their daughter but they are encouraged to feel more confident about their ability to deal with difficult situations that might arise. The therapist facilitates negotiations between parents and daughter so that she can start to take more responsibility for her mealtime behaviour. If there are any significant problems, Phase 1 is revisited. Family concerns and issues that have had to take a back seat are now discussed with the therapist and healthy family functioning is emphasised.

Phase 3: Adolescent issues and termination

This phase commences once the adolescent reaches 90–100% of ideal weight and has appropriate control over food intake. The focus is taken off the re-feeding process, and the adolescent's identity and individuality is explored in detail for the first time. Throughout Phase 1 and 2 the therapist has helped the family to restructure more appropriate boundaries so that their child can now continue to develop individuality in an appropriate way. Her healthy development had previously been impeded by the control exerted by the anorexia. A wide variety of adolescent issues are explored and worked through with the family, including separation, peer relationships and sexuality. The parents are also encouraged to give up attitudes and skills that were appropriate at earlier stages in their child's life and to spend more time together as a couple. If particular problems arise the parents are advised to seek couple therapy in order to deal with their own issues. It is not always the case that a strong parenting team leads to a happier marriage (Maudsley Parents, 2013; Rhodes, 2003).

CONCLUSION

Now that you have read this chapter and learnt some of the key ideas behind different therapeutic interventions you should have an understanding that whatever the approach used the relationship with the young person and their family is paramount.

A child, young person or family must feel that they are supported, listened to and respected by workers, therapists and the team and organisation within which they are being seen. Therapists and practitioners must have faith and hope that all families, children and young people have the capacity for change in this window of opportunity.

REFERENCES

Allen, G. (2011) *Early Intervention: Smart Investment, Massive Savings*. Available from: www. gov.uk/government/uploads/system/uploads/attachment_data/file/61012/earlyintervention-smartinvestment.pdf (accessed August 2013).

Association for Play Therapy (2013) *Play Therapy Defined*. Available from: www.a4pt.org/ ps.playtherapy.cfm (accessed August 2013).

Beck, A.T. (1976) *Cognitive Therapy and Emotional Disorders*. London: Penguin Books.

Bell, D. (2000) Who is Killing What or Whom? Some Notes on the Internal Phemenology of Suicide. *Psychoanalytic Psychotherapy*, 15 (1): 21–37.

Berman, A. and Jobes, D. (1991) *Adolescent Suicide: Assessment and Intervention*. Washington, DC: American Psychological Association.

Bonham, P. (2004) *Communicating as a Mental Health Carer*. Cheltenham: Nelson Thornes.

Briggs, S. (2002) Working with the Risk of Suicide in Young People. *Journal of Social Work Practice*, 16 (2): 135–48.

British Association for Counselling and Psychotherapy (2013) *School-based Counselling: What is it and Why we Need it*. Available from: www.bacp.co.uk/admin/structure/files/ pdf/11791_sbc_may2013.pdf (accessed August 2013).

Burnham, J. (1986) *Family Therapy*. Hove: Routledge.

Burstow, P., Rt Hon. (2012) IAPT for Children and Young People (press release). Department of Health. Available from: www.gov.uk/government/news/16-july-2012-paul-burstow-iapt-for-children-and-young-people (accessed August 2013).

CAMHS (2008) *Child and Adolescent Mental Health Services Review*. Available from: www. bacp.co.uk/admin/structure/files/pdf/11791_sbc_may2013.pdf (accessed August 2013).

Campbell, D. and Hale, R. (1991) Suicidal Acts. In Holmes, J. (ed.) *Textbook of Psychotherapy in Psychiatric Practice*. London: Churchill Livingstone, pp. 287–306.

Cecchin, G. (1987) Hypothesising, Circularity and Neutrality Revisited: An Invitation to Curiosity. *Family Process*, 26 (4): 405–13.

Cecchin, G. (1992) Constucting Therapeutic Possibilities. In McNamee, S. Gergen and K. J. (eds), *Therapy as a Social Construction* London: Sage.

CYP IAPT (Children and Young People's Improving Access to Psychological Therapies) (2012) *Newsletter*, December. Available from: www.iapt.nhs.uk/silo/files/cyp-iapt-newsletter-3-december-2012.pdf (accessed August 2013).

Department for Education and Skills (2003) *Every Child Matters*. Available from: www. education.gov.uk/publications/standard/publicationDetail/Page1/DfES%200672%20 2003 (accessed August 2013).

Department of Health (2013) *Annual Report of the Chief Medical Officer Our Children Deserve Better: Prevention Pays*. Available from: www.gov.uk/government/uploads/system/ uploads/attachments_data/file/255237/2901304_CMO_complete_low_res_accessible.pdf (accessed January 2014).

Department of Health and Department for Education (2004) *National Service Framework for Children, Young People and Maternity Services* Available from: www.gov.uk/government/uploads/system/uploads/attachment_data/file/199952/National_Service_Framework_for_Children_Young_People_and_Maternity_Services_-_Core_Standards.pdf (accessed August 2013).

Dogra, N., Parkin, A., Gale, F. and Frake, C. (2009) *A Multidisciplinary Handbook of Child and Adolescent Mental Health for Front-line Professionals*, 2nd edn. London: Jessica Kingsley.

Fraiberg, S. (1980) *Clinical Studies in Infant Mental Health*. New York: Basic Books.

Fuggle, P. Dunsmuir, S. and Curry, V. (2013) *CBT with Children, Young People and Families*. London: Sage.

Hedges, F. (2005) *An Introduction to Systemic Therapy with Individuals*. London: Sage.

HM Government (2011) *No Health Without Mental Health: A Cross-government Mental Health Outcomes Strategy for People of All Ages*. Available from: www.gov.uk/government/uploads/system/uploads/attachment_data/file/213761/dh_124058.pdf (accessed August 2013).

Hopper, L. (2006) *Counselling and Psychotherapy with Children and Adolescents*. Basingstoke: Palgrave Macmillan.

Jones, A. (2006) Levels of Change in Parent–Infant Psychotherapy. *Journal of Child Psychotherapy*, 32 (3): 295–311.

Jones, E. (1993) *Family Systems Therapy*. Chichester: John Wiley.

Landreth, G. (2002) *Play Therapy: The Art of the Relationship*, 2nd edn. Hove: Routledge.

Landreth, G. (2012) *Child Centered Play Therapy DVD Review*. Routledge Therapy. Available from: www.youtube.com/watch?v=JIMWOOlR_9g (accessed August 2013).

Loy, J., Merry, S., Hetrick, S. and Stasiak, K. (2012) Atypical Antipsychotics for Disruptive Behaviour Disorders in Children and Youths (Review). *The Cochrane Collaboration*, 12 September.

McLeod, J. (2003) *An Introduction to Counselling*, 3rd edn. Maidenhead: Open University Press.

Maudsley Parents (2013) *Family-based Treatment of Anorexia Nervosa: The Maudsley Approach*. Available from: www.maudsleyparents.org/whatismaudsley.html (accessed August 2013).

Mental Health Foundation (2006) *Truth Hurts: Report of the National Inquiry into Self Harm among Young People*. Available from: www.mentalhealth.org.uk/content/assets/PDF/publications/truth_hurts.pdf?view=Standard (accessed August 2013).

Miller, L. (2008) The Relation of Infant Observation to Clinical Practice in an Under-fives Counselling Service. In Emanuel, L. and Bradley, E. (eds) *'What Can the Matter Be?' Therapeutic Interventions with Parents, Infants and Young Children: The Work of the Tavistock Clinic Under-Fives Service*. London: Karnac, pp. 38–53.

National Institute for Clinical Excellence (2004a) *Eating Disorders: Core Interventions in the Treatment and Management of Anorexia Nervosa, Bulimia Nervosa, and Related Eating Disorders*. Available from: www.nice.org.uk/nicemedia/live/10932/29220/29220.pdf (accessed August 2013).

National Institute for Clinical Excellence (2004b) *Self-harm: The Short-term Physical and Psychological Management and Secondary Prevention of Self-harm in Primary and Secondary Care*. Available from: www.nice.org.uk/nicemedia/pdf/CG016NICEguideline.pdf (accessed August 2013).

National Institute for Clinical Excellence (2005) *Depression in Children and Young People*. Available from: www.nice.org.uk/nicemedia/live/10970/29856/29856.pdf (accessed August 2013).

National Institute for Clinical Excellence (2006) *Bipolar Disorder: The Management of Bipolar Disorder in Adults, Children and Adolescents in Primary and Secondary Care.* Available from: www.nice.org.uk/nicemedia/pdf/CG38niceguideline.pdf (accessed August 2013).

National Institute for Clinical Excellence (2008) *Attention Deficit Hyperactivity Disorder: Diagnosis and Management of ADHD in Children, Young People and Adults.* Available from: www.nice.org.uk/nicemedia/live/12061/42059/42059.pdf (accessed August 2013).

National Institute for Clinical Excellence (2013) *Social Anxiety Disorder: Recognition, Assessment and Treatment.* Available from: www.nice.org.uk/nicemedia/live/14168/63868/63868.pdf (accessed August 2013).

Neenan, M. and Dryden, W. (2006) *Cognitive Therapy in a Nutshell.* London: Sage.

Norton, L. (2011) *Innovative Interventions in Child and Adolescent Mental Health.* London: Routledge.

Palazzoli S., Boscolo, L., Cecchin, G. and Prata, G. (1980) Hypothesizing-Circularity-Neutrality: Three Guidelines for the Conductor of the Session. *Family Process*, 19 (1): 3–12.

PbR CAMHS (2013) *CAMHS Payment by Results Pilot Project.* Available from: pbrcamhs. org/ (accessed September 2013).

Pozzi-Monzo, M., Lee, A. and Likierman, M. (2011) From Reactive to Reflective: Evidence for Shifts in Parents' State of Mind during Brief Under-fives Psychoanalytic Psychotherapy. *Clinical Child Psychology and Psychiatry*, 17 (1): 151–64.

Prevatt, F. (1999) Milan Systemic Theory. In Lawson, D. and Prevatt, F. (eds) *Casebook in Family Therapy.* Belmont, CA: Brooks Cole, pp. 189–209.

Prever, M. (2010) *Counselling and Supporting Children and Young People: A Person-centred Approach.* London: Sage.

Rhodes, P. (2003) The Maudsley Model of Family Therapy for Children and Adolescents with Anorexia Nervosa: Theory, Clinical Practice, and Empirical Support. *Australian and New Zealand Journal of Family Therapy*, 24 (4): 191–8.

Rivett, M. and Street, E. (2009) *Family Therapy 100 Key Concepts and Techniques.* Hove: Routledge.

Rogers, C. (1957) The Necessary and Sufficient Conditions for Therapeutic Change. *Journal of Consulting Psychology*, 21: 95–103.

Royal College of Psychiatrists (2012) *PbR CAMHS Consultation Document, CAMHS PbR Project.* Available from: www.rcpsych.ac.uk/pdf/CAMHS%20PbR%20Consultation.pdf (accessed September 2013).

Sanders, D. and Wills, F. (2005) *Cognitive Therapy: An Introduction*, 2nd edn. London: Sage.

Stallard, P. (2002) *Think Good, Feel Good: A Cognitive Behaviour Therapy Workbook for Children and Young People.* Chichester: Wiley.

Stallard, P. (2009) *Anxiety: Cognitive Behaviour Therapy with Children and Young People.* Hove: Routledge.

Wohl, M. (1995) Depression and Guilt. In Laufer, M. (ed.) *The Suicidal Adolescent.* London: Karnac, pp. 29–34.

Yalom, I. (1980) *Existential Psychotherapy.* New York: Basic Books.

7

GROUP WORK WITH CHILDREN, YOUNG PEOPLE AND FAMILIES

BRIONY WILLIAMS

Overview

- Setting up and starting groups
- Group process
- Types of groups
- Theoretical framework
- Group facilitation and leadership
- Factors that influence facilitation
- Group structure
- Nurturing inclusion
- Strategies for dealing with problems in groups

INTRODUCTION

Group work is an effective way of working with people of all ages who have similar problems and needs. Children and young people are used to being in groups; they live their lives within family groups, school groups and friendship groups. Group work can provide young people with the opportunity to practise important and useful communication and relationship skills. Groups are a natural opportunity for socialisation and support; the communication and relationship skills that develop can be transferred to young people's lives outside the group (Lindsay and Orton, 2011; Rose, 1998). This chapter develops the knowledge of planning and facilitating group activities and techniques for working with children, young people and their families.

There may be pressure from managers to run groups because they are seen as a cost-effective way of helping a larger number of children. One advantage when comparing group work over individual work is that groups can be less time-consuming than seeing people individually. However we need to be aware that the time also includes planning, support and evaluation. Unfortunately some workers are wary of groups. Potential group workers may worry about the responsibility of group planning and group facilitation; running a group will involve a lot of planning and thought; it is not as straightforward as arranging to see people individually. Benson (2010) points out that the importance of planning cannot be emphasised enough: many groups do not get off the ground due to a lack of planning and organisation before the group started. When groups are embedded in practice and there is a system in place for planning them, they tend to run smoothly and the benefits for group members are clear.

Prever (2011: 11) suggests that working with children and young people is different to working with adults; he says when 'working with children we are working with potential, with futures, with transition, with growth and becoming'. Campion (1991) recommends workers in groups for children and young people have a good understanding of child development. Group work is about problem solving, offering more perspectives to assist personal growth and finding solutions. It is also a way for young people to put their problems to one side by helping others, which then provides increased feelings of self-worth (Lindsay and Orton, 2011). Hamori and Hodi (1996) suggest that group work can offer children and adolescents a powerful therapeutic arena in which they can explore and experiment with a range of different situations that mirror the delicate and often difficult dynamics that operate within families and other intimate relationships. Participants in groups often experience a sense of belonging, with support from people who are coping with similar problems. Many of the people who attended the groups that I facilitated said that the main benefit at first was finding out that they were not alone. Strong relationships can develop in a group between young people and the facilitators of the group and more importantly their peers. A group for children can be an opportunity to develop a 'self which is more flexible and robust than a relationship with one other person alone' (Luxmoore, 2008: 52). Some of our best and worst experiences will have been in groups. Groups can be about being liked, accepted and respected but it is important to remember that they can also be about being persecuted and rejected (Luxmoore, 2008: 53). Groups can mirror the wider social environment so they are able to promote change which could be more difficult in individual counselling (Geldard and Geldard, 2008: 90). Groups work because people have the capacity to learn from their experiences and from each other. Westergaard (2009: 6) agrees, stating that a group is made up of individuals with shared needs who will benefit from the opportunity to work with, and learn from others in order to develop skills, knowledge and attitudes.

SETTING UP AND STARTING GROUPS

Activity

What do you imagine are the fears of a 16-year-old who has been asked to go to a group to discuss their problems? The following list are some of the comments from past group members.

- Fear of being seen as different by others who have not been told to go to the group.
- Fears about the size of the group.
- Fear of being the 'worst'.
- Fear of other group members behaviour.
- Fears linked to their experience of groups at school.
- Fear of being rejected by other group members.
- Fears of being judged.
- Fear of confessing embarrassing experiences or thoughts.

Children are naturally in groups at school and at home and often what they experience will influence how they expect to be treated. For example a young person who is referred to a group which aims to combat anxiety and boost self-esteem will most likely be coming to the group having had negative experiences at school or other settings. If you are running a support group for parents, experience of past groups such as school are still influential. Some of our fears of entering a group originate from our early experience; memories of being picked on or laughed at in school. Teachers who criticised you in front of the class, other children laughing at you when you made a mistake, not feeling 'good enough' and feeling left out are common problems and it is important that these fears are acknowledged.

Cooper and Tiknaz (2007: 16) found some students are very quiet and withdrawn and some excitable and disruptive when they first attend a group. The group facilitator is responsible for ensuring that the start of the group reassures participants that this current group experience will be positive and supportive. I remember the person who supervised me when I ran groups saying that the first five minutes of the group set the tone. I have often remembered those words and agree that the planning before the group and the way you start your first group are very important. Luxmoore (2008: 59) agrees, 'the eventual quality of a group's experience depends very much on the quality of its beginning'.

Preparing clients for a group

The preparation for a group starts weeks before the group commences and includes assessment of clients, letter writing or phone calls, booking a room, buying resources and finally setting up the room. I was almost obsessional about the room preparation, making sure that the chairs were all the same and that there were enough for all group members and they were arranged in a perfect circle with the same gap in between each one. This was partly because of my anxiety in preparation for a new group but important too as the new group members need to feel that they are all equal, that there is no rush for the more comfortable chair.

Meeting and assessing group members

It is good practice to meet all group members prior to the group starting. In therapy groups all group members should be assessed by the group facilitators before they come to the group. There needs to be some thought as to the individual's suitability for the group and whether they will cope with a group setting. Children are assessed to rule out causal factors which might need to be addressed differently and 'the group is not a substitute for primary needs such as child protection, medical needs, good parenting and good education' (Drost and Bayley, 2001: 22). Another aspect of this meeting is that the potential group member needs to assess you and decide if the group is right for them. You may be tempted to avoid this step if you are working in a close team and take other co-workers' referral without meeting the person to assess their suitability for the group yourself. The group facilitators know the aims and objectives of their group well and it is only them who can make the assessment of an individual's needs and capabilities to check that the group is a good fit. Groups may be harmful for some young people; one young person may be different from the rest of the people who are coming to the group (Lindsay and Orton, 2011). The first interview is also an assessment that the individuals who have been referred have similar needs, are of a similar developmental age and have the ability to understand the concepts being discussed. However this is dependent on the type of group that is being run; in an activity-based group the developmental level is less important than in an educational group or a cognitive behavioural group.

The assessment or introductory interview is also the start of your relationship with the individual and a chance to build rapport; children, young people and parents alike are more likely to turn up for the frightening first group if they have met you. Drost and Bayley (2001) assess children before they come to the group in order to get to know them. Geldard and Geldard (2001) suggest that this step is necessary to avoid a catastrophe, a dysfunctional group or a major conflict; they also state that screening or introductory interviews will diminish the prospect of children dropping out. Luxmoore (2008) describes meeting with six young people individually for a while before the first group was planned, talking with them about the group which they agreed to join even though they had mixed feelings. At the start of the first session he had some awareness of the likely behaviours and defences of the young people.

Pre-group assessment measures

Evaluating the effectiveness of any intervention is increasingly important. There are standardised measures which would need to be used if the group outcomes are to be appropriately assessed. It is possible to create non-standardised measures and self-evaluation questionnaires based on the objectives of the group.

GROUP PROCESS

Group process is about how groups develop and change over time (Geldard and Geldard, 2001). The process is not to do with the aims and goals of the group or the activities chosen. Group process is more about the interpersonal relationships of the group members and how these change and develop over the course of the group sessions. Awareness of the group process is useful as it will influence the way you set up, facilitate and how you finish the group. Group process can be influenced by the activities you choose and how you facilitate the activities, but it also happens regardless of the aims and goals of the group. The chosen theoretical perspective can make sense of the group process and group dynamics; each theoretical perspective will have a different perspective for viewing the process and dynamics. To simplify group process it is about the beginning of the group, the middle of the group and the ending of the group.

The most influential theorist discussing group process is Tuckman (1965). He examined how groups develop over time and saw a general pattern. Tuckman (1965) said that groups go through stages of forming, storming, norming and performing. More recently, a fifth and final stage was added, called mourning or adjourning.

Geldard and Geldard (2001) describe a similar four-stage model for groups with children which covers the actual group experience: forming, storming, norming, mourning with the addition of preparation (before the group starts) and closure (working with children when the group ends).

Beginning

This stage is inevitably at the start of a group, however, it may also happen if several new people arrive at the same time to an established group. It is quite normal for group leaders and children to feel anxious in the first session; Geldard and Geldard (2001) suggest this anxiety is useful as it provides the energy required for success. I am not sure if I ever commenced the first session of a group without being aware of my increased anxiety. I was usually over-prepared and found myself rearranging the chairs so that the gaps between them were equidistant. Luxmoore (2008: 52) shares his anxieties: 'I am pretty sure about what we're going to do and I have various strategies in my head in case things go wrong. But I am still nervous.' He shares his preparations for a self-esteem group: 'The room is as prepared as it can be. My hope is that a calmly organised room will make for a calmly organised group.'

The members of the group are new to each other. They're unsure of each other and unsure of the purpose of the group. Their first responsibility is to become a group and find an identity. Individuals are anxious and looking for direction and rely heavily on the facilitator or group leader. Luxmoore (2008) recommends a structure so that the children know what to do so that they do not do anything stupid and make a fool of themselves. Children need the group leader to be a leader so that they do not have to take over and run things for themselves.

However, if a group leader is too directive at this stage it may result in group members only relating to them and not forming together. This will slow down the process of achieving cohesion. The leader may be challenged as group members become more familiar with each other. Personality clashes and differences of opinion are likely. This part of the process is called storming. A child may decide not to turn up for a group. Luxmoore (2008) discusses what to do with the empty chair in this scenario and argues that it is important to leave the empty chair in the group and discuss the decision with the rest of the group. The atmosphere of the group has changed and feels uncomfortable. Children may be argumentative or resistant, apathetic or silent. These problems in groups will be discussed in more detail later in the chapter. It is likely that a scapegoat will emerge and subgroups may develop. A scapegoat is someone who is perceived to be different from the rest of the group and the problems of the group are transferred to the scapegoat rather than the group as a whole. This may be the leader because participants find it easier to blame the leader for all of the problems within the group.

Luxmoore (2008) describes a boy who is silent in the group and this behaviour could easily be perceived by the other group members as refusal to enter the group rather than anxiety about disclosure. The boy may be scapegoated by the other group members because they are also uneasy about their own disclosures, they would feel more comfortable without him. Pre-existing patterns of behaviour linked to early relationships, experiences and familiar ways of relating to others often become mirrored in group settings. Often in families we are unwittingly assigned roles which may be played out in the other groups we are part of. A child who is regarded as difficult in the family, the problem child, might well become the scapegoat in the new group. It is a familiar role, the child understands the rules, role and the interactions, sometimes actively encouraging them.

Although storming is an uncomfortable stage it is one of the most important. It could be argued that we never truly have an honest and trusting relationship unless we allow ourselves to disagree. It is important for the leader to remain calm and grounded, displaying strength and patience towards the group members and surviving the attacks without retaliating during this stage (Geldard and Geldard, 2001; Luxmoore, 2008). If effectively managed by the group facilitator, the group process models a secure base and can be a powerful opportunity for positive change.

Middle

During these stages the group begins to find mutual direction and a consensus emerges partly because of the creative ideas which have been thrown around during the storming stage and partly because group members want to move away from the storming stage. This stage feels more harmonious and less superficial than the form-ing stage. This stage can feel complacent but if the storming stage has been allowed to occur, the group can feel positive and intimate. The group starts to fully apply themselves to the task. They get on with the work that needs to be done. They may take on new activities and because they know each other quite well they feel safe to take on different roles and activities.

Ending

It is important not to ignore or miss out this stage. The last session needs to contain an evaluation of the group as a whole and involve all group members, acknowledg-ing that the group is ending. Group members will need to say gooodbye to each other within the group setting. This stage may happen when members of the group leave or new members join. Group members will look back and review events from the past and will look forward with excitement and fear to future challenges. It is natural at this stage for group members to experience negative feelings for the group as a way of coping and feeling better about leaving them. You need to pre-pare for the end of the group at the start.

THE GROUP STRUCTURE

The structure of each session should have a warm up, main activity and wind down or beginning, middle and end. Westergaard (2009) explains stage 1, the beginning: welcomes and introductions; stage 2, the middle: engage with the activities to explore the topic in more detail; and stage 3, the end: summarise the main points and plan actions.

Introductions

At the start of the first group introduce the group facilitators and include some background information and their past experience running groups. The group members need to feel confident that the group facilitators are qualified and expe-rienced enough to see them through the group process. Ask the group members to introduce themselves and say that they do not have to go into too much detail. In the first group it is a good idea to ask the group members to form pairs to discuss an aspect of the group or what they are hoping to get from the group. This exercise allows group members to get to know one other person a little more deeply and start to find common ground and make connections. It is important to invite early participation as group members will be worried about not speaking in the group and the longer the group goes on without some contribution the higher the level of anxiety. It is good to have a pairs exercise to encourage clients to interact directly with each other rather than all of the communication going through the group leader. Use activities which foster cooperation and a sense of commonality. Try separating the group into two smaller groups to share and write ideas down on flipchart paper to use as a prop for discussion.

Environmental information

Group members need to know where the toilets are, what to do and where to go in case of a fire alarm and the arrangements for a break and refreshment facilities. Giving out this type of information early in the first session can help allay fears and provide a structure.

Group aims

Group members need to know the aims and goals of the group and a little information about some of the content of the group and the normal structure of the group. If age appropriate give a handout noting the number of sessions, the timing of the sessions and roughly the content and goals of each session; this provides structure and reduces fear. The group facilitators believe that the clients will benefit from the group and it is important to explain how group therapy works and to give examples of group exercises. The group facilitators are selling the idea of the group for personal growth and change and may need to explain how group therapy can address individual problems.

Rules and boundaries

Ask group members to own and make rules for the group and this is better done towards the end of the first group. Luxmoore (2008) points out that young people may find it difficult to think of the rules they make for themselves before they know about the aims of the group and why rules may be needed. Giving young people the responsibility for regulating their own behaviour is a gradual process (Luxmoore, 2008: 64). In the first session the group leader may need to give guidelines of how to participate in groups and how behaviour will be managed. Setting ground rules enables young people to become active participants (Westergaard, 2009). Rules could be written on a large piece of flipchart paper and pinned on the wall each week or typed up and then given out to group members the following week. The following list are some of the rules that group members suggest:

- Respect the need for confidentiality.
- Everybody is important.
- Try not to judge people's behaviour.
- It's important to turn up to the group.
- You can make mistakes.
- It's OK not to know the answers.
- It's OK to ask for help.
- Turn mobile phones off.

TYPES OF GROUPS

Here are some that you may have listed:

- Your first family group
- Wider family groups including grandparents, aunts, uncles and cousins
- School groups
- Peer groups
- Organised groups for young people such as Brownies, Scouts, sports groups, activity groups
- New family groups we create as we grow up
- University groups, sports groups or political groups
- Therapy groups as participants.

These groups could be organised into natural groups that you belonged to and organised groups set up for a purpose (Douglas, 2000).

Preston-Shoot (2007) states that an individual's childhood and later experiences are recreated as emotional tensions in the context of the group. I have found this affected me as a facilitator of the group; I have to rein in my inclination to take control and do everything myself. Group facilitators can use methods and activities to identify disturbing conflicts from the past and bring them into awareness so that the young person can try out new ways of relating to others.

A group leader must be aware of the group members' needs and therefore the type and purpose of the group. If the group leader's ideas are hazy the group members will be uncertain. Benson (2010) points out that group leaders who start groups without being clear about their reasons for using group work and without adequate planning are likely to have problems. Where the focus of the session is not decided at the outset, the session is likely to be messy and at best will be unlikely to achieve positive outcomes for the young people involved (Westergaard, 2009). Group members pick up on the lack of planning and feel unsafe. My experience running a group is that if people feel unsafe in the group they stop attending. This is a basic fight and flight instinct; when we feel afraid we feel like running away or avoiding the situation that makes us feel fear. The impact of feeling unsafe in a group can also result in children or young people feeling that they do not trust the leader, creating the capacity for the children to sabotage or disrupt the group. Individual attachment styles will influence behaviour in groups. A child or young person's attachment style will be replicated in a group setting as it would be in any arena of human relationships.

Table 7.1 gives an outline of different types of groups.

Table 7.1   Example of different types of groups in CAMHS

Type of group	Description of group	Examples of groups for children and young people
CAMHS Tier 3 and 4 groups Therapy groups/ group psychotherapy	The groups usually take place in a residential unit or in the community and are run by health or social care professionals such as nurses, occupational therapists, psychologists and social workers. The groups target children who have a mental health problem (Geldard and Geldard, 2001). These groups have an overlying theoretical approach and it is vital when running this level of group that the facilitators are trained and have a clear understanding of the theoretical model and child and adolescent mental health.	The groups may include cognitive therapy groups, e.g. anxiety management groups, anger management groups, social skills groups and assertion training. Hearing voices groups and social confidence groups for young people with psychosis. Psychotherapy and psychodynamic groups can include transactional analysis groups, gestalt groups, psychodrama groups and projective art groups.
CAMHS Tiers 2, 3 and 4 Counselling groups	Helpful for children who are finding it difficult to cope with life's challenges (Geldard and Geldard, 2001). They are useful for resolving problems and preventing the development of problems.	There are various approaches that may be used. Geldard and Geldard (2001) suggest an experiential approach. Some therapists use a humanistic approach and others use a cognitive behavioural approach.

Type of group	Description of group	Examples of groups for children and young people
CAMHS Tiers 1 and above Psycho-education groups or educational groups	Psycho-education groups focus on gaining information and knowledge and tend to be more structured than other groups. They help children learn and develop healthy constructs and therefore change attitudes and behaviours. They use strategies from an educational and cognitive behavioural approach.	Drug and alcohol education group with the aim of increasing young people's awareness of the psychological, physical and biological effects.
CAMHS Tiers 1 and above Personal growth groups, youth groups	Some of the groups in the community have aims to increase social interaction; to help participants to gain social contact. The groups are often open groups with no set beginning or end session.	Youth centres running pottery groups, art groups, cooking groups, budgeting groups, indoor and outdoor groups.
Personal Learning and Development Groups (Westergaard, 2009)	Attend to personal issues, focusing on each individual's personal and development needs, in a group setting (Westergaard, 2009).	
CAMHS Tier 1 and above Developmental skills groups	Group aims to work on skills development where group members work to increase life skills or academic skills.	Activity groups may involve cookery, pottery, sport and brain gym.
CAMHS Tier 1 and above Support groups	Support groups may include gaining support for an illness or a loss such as coping with the death of a loved one. These groups are most likely open groups where group members can join at any time and participate in as many sessions as they need to. It is common for people to dip in and out of the group as they feel the need rather than commit to a set number of sessions.	Young carers groups. Gaining support regarding a condition such as diabetes, ADHD or Asperger's; these may be run by professionals with knowledge of the condition. Bereavement groups. Crisis intervention groups in a school setting following a crisis or disaster (Rose, 1998).

Although it is usual to run the groups for people of a similar developmental age it is also possible that you may run a group and include children and adults together, for example a support group for parents and children where the aim is to improve relationships. Some groups can be a mixture of two of the types of groups shown in the table, although it is unlikely that you would mix skill development groups with psychotherapy groups as the aims are too diverse.

Groups can be long- or short-term, they are usually time-limited but could be ongoing (Preston-Shoot, 2007). Ongoing groups could be open to new group members; time-limited groups are usually closed groups with the same group of people starting on group one and expected to stay for the duration. Open groups can offer ongoing support; however group members may be come dependent and not seek support in other social networks. The type of activity chosen within the group will change dependent on the type of group. For example at the most practical level the activity may be to use art with young children; the type of group may be a skill development group and the goals are to increase the amount of time the children are able to stay involved and concentrate on the task. At a different level, an art group may be used to increase social interaction. The difference in this type of group is that the facilitator would be less directive and the young people would make decisions about what they want to do. Lloyd et al. (2008) advocate the active involvement of young people with psychosis in the process of collaborative goal setting. This process of joint decision making develops useful communication and relationship skills. Art may also be used as a support group where the art may be directed towards a topic that is common to all participants and discussion would take place throughout the group. At the deepest level, art would be used in a psychotherapy group where the young people may work in relative silence painting a picture of an aspect of their life. The participants take it in turns to talk about their picture. An example of a possible subject is 'how I see myself and how others see me'. Creative media such as clay, music, drama and creative writing can be used in all of these types of groups and at these different levels. The type of group will influence the aims and goals of the group and therefore the content of the group and the activities chosen. It is important to decide on the type and aims of the group having assessed the needs of the group members to ensure a good fit.

Age

Age is an important consideration when thinking about the type of group; it is also important that participants have similar capabilities and are at a similar developmental stage. When discussing a group for 6- 8-year-old children coping with parents' separation Rose (1998) suggests group leaders concentrate on improving mood and dispelling guilt and confusion. Group work with this age focuses on concrete discussion of events; the group is mostly directed and prepared by the group leaders. In an older age group who are more aware of social situations and meaning and can think about others' perspectives, children are aware of and measure themselves against social standards set by adults and influenced by peers (Geldard and Geldard, 2001). At this stage children may isolate themselves from others and be secretive. Conflict resolution strategies are suggested and constructive ways of working with anger because at this age loyalty conflicts and anger were found to be the major issue (Rose, 1998). Developmental age is affected by mental health problems such as depression and psychosis. Young people suffering from psychosis show significant impairment in many areas of social functioning (Lloyd et al., 2008).

THEORETICAL FRAMEWORK

A theoretical framework is a way of understanding the individual group member's problems and relationships. It is also a way of constructing the group activities and directing the facilitator responses. A lack of clarity about the theoretical framework can create confusion and anxiety for group members (Preston-Shoot, 2007). It is important for group facilitators to be trained and have a good level of knowledge in the theory before leading a group. Table 7.2 describes the types of groups that might be run within different theoretical frameworks.

Table 7.2 CAMHS groups according to theoretical framework

Theoretical framework	Type of group	Description of group
Psychological		
Psychodynamic Tiers 3 and 4	Any type of creative group, e.g. an art group, pottery group, music group, creative writing group	'Childhoods and later experiences are recreated as emotional tensions in the context of the group and its leader' (Preston Shoot, 2007: 64).
Humanistic Tiers 1–4	Self-esteem group Personal learning and development groups (Westergaard, 2009)	'Emphasise human emotional development and the power of the group to facilitate the release of feelings and the achievement of personal growth' (Preston Shoot, 2007: 64).
Cognitive Tiers 2–4	Coping with feelings group Improve your mood group	Understanding the relationship between feelings and thoughts; analysing deep-seated beliefs and their impact on self-image.
Cognitive behavioural group Tiers 1–4	Anxiety management group	Understanding the interconnection of thinking and feeling on behaviours. Understanding the physical signs of anxiety, explaining fight and flight and helping group members challenge negative thinking patterns and set realistic goals.
Behavioural Tiers 1–4	Social skills group Domestic skills group Budgeting skills group	Using positive reinforcement, and sometimes negative reinforcement to shape behaviour. Setting behavioural goals for change. Role play is also used to practise new behaviours in a safe group environment. Relaxation may be used to reduce physiological symptoms of anxiety.

(Continued)

Table 7.2   (Continued)

Theoretical framework	Type of group	Description of group
Transactional analysis	Coping with feelings group Healthy relationships group	Explaining transactional analysis theory to group members and using the theory to help analyse group members' patterns of transactions with themselves (intra-personal communication) and others (interpersonal communication).
Sociological		
Systemic Tiers 1 and 2	Youth group	'Views the group as a system and each member as a subsystem within it and the group as part of a wider network' (Preston Shoot, 2007: 64).
Feminist Tiers 1 and 2	Domestic violence group	Challenges the view of women as subordinate and promotes their ability to take control of their lives (Preston Shoot, 2007: 65).
Educational		
Personal learning and development groups (Westergaard, 2009) Tiers 1 and 2	Transition from primary to secondary school group A group for prospective foster parents	Offer information and impart skills through instruction (Preston Shoot, 2007: 53). Introducing group members to new ways of carrying out a new task. Preparing group members for new experiences and challenges.

GROUP FACILITATION/LEADERSHIP

The type of group and the theoretical framework that underpins the group will often determine whether the group is facilitated or led. A facilitator is less directive and less structured than a leader. Preston-Shoot (2007) describes a facilitator as being concerned with process and good communication and being neutral about the content and having no stake in decisions. A facilitator puts in a lot of preparation before the group to make the group easier for group members and allow the group to flow. They assist groups as they work together towards achieving a goal. The group members are responsible for the results from their efforts; however the facilitators remain alert to group dynamics and create a safe space for discussion. For group members, especially children and young people, the facilitator's refusal to take charge could be frustrating; this may be necessary and integral to the aim of the group in order for the young people to take charge and develop skills.

Leadership styles

The personality of the group leader, the theoretical framework used and the type of group and the stage of the group will have an impact on the leadership style. The leader may need to be more directive at the start of a group and be able to relax towards the middle of the group and again take more control towards the end of the group to manage closure. The most effective leaders will also be skilled facilitators. If you are running a creative activity group for young children you will need to be more directive; Geldard and Geldard (2001) suggest an authoritarian approach when running a group for children who have ADHD. An authoritarian leader thinks they know what is best for the group, they will direct with the conviction that what they think and have planned is right; in some circumstances such as a crisis this may be the most appropriate style. This style produces the greatest output but can create hostility, low morale, poor quality and dependence (Lewin et al., 1939). Also at this highly directive and controlling end of the scale is the autocratic style. Some group leaders want to control the group but do not want to appear autocratic so are manipulative in style. This is when the leader wishes to dominate the group but also takes into account the views of others as they try and sell the situation to others in the group.

The behaviours in the middle of the range of leadership styles are democratic; they seek collaboration and participation in decision making. Lewin et al. (1939) found that the democratic style is the most effective overall. Cole (2005) further divides and discusses differences within democratic leadership:

> *Directive:* defines the group, selects activities and structures designed to be therapeutically appropriate to specific service user groups. This is an effective approach for groups who have difficulties with decision making and problem solving.

> *Facilitative:* openly discusses the purpose and function of the group and encourages the group to make decisions with their guidance. This approach assumes a certain level of self-awareness and intelligence and an ability to develop insight.

> *Adviser:* the most passive of the leadership styles. This approach is limited to the highest function groups. Advice or expertise is offered but no structure is provided. The motivation comes from the group itself.

At the less directive end Lewin et al. (1939) describe laissez-faire or permissive leadership where group members are left alone to do as they please, which produces independence but poor morale; however, it can be effective in situations where group members are highly skilled, motivated and capable of working on their own. Children may find the lack of boundaries with this style difficult.

Activity

Reflect about what could go wrong for you when leading a group.

For a new leader directive leadership feels safer and less threatening than the less struc-tured styles of leadership. At the same time new group leaders may be in conflict, feel discomfort about authority and fear of losing control. Part of the exercise in group leadership is the exercise of control (Brown, 1994, cited in Doel, 2007: 99). Heron (1989, cited in Burnard, 1990: 181) identified six dimensions of facilitation style:

> *Directive or non-directive:* the type of group and the overarching theoretical framework will influence how much the facilitator directs the group. A behavioural group tends to be directed whereas a humanistic group tends to be less directed.

> *Interpretive or non-interpretive:* the facilitator offers interpretations of behaviour in psy-choanalytical groups and transactional analysis groups but not in behavioural or task groups.

> *Confronting or non-confronting:* the facilitator needs to challenge the group carefully to encourage a different way of thinking and to understand the impact of an irrational belief in a cognitive behavioural group.

> *Cathartic or non-cathartic:* the facilitator encourages an emotional release of feelings in a psychotherapy group but would not actively encourage it when working with an educa-tional frame of reference.

> *Structuring or un-structuring:* in an anxiety management group exercises have been pre-selected and planned by the group leaders. In an art project group for young people the facilitators would encourage the group participants to choose the activities and create the structure.

> *Disclosing or non-disclosing:* in an anxiety management or coping with feelings or self-esteem group it is a good idea for the facilitator to model appropriate self-disclosure. It is not advisable to disclose current unresolved problems or issues. The main aim is for the group members to gain help and the only reason you should share is to assist their under-standing, not for you to gain help from the group. In strict psychoanalytical groups the therapist shares very little of their self.

FACTORS THAT INFLUENCE FACILITATION

Choosing the activities

The activities planned are integral to the success and enjoyment of the group. They should be meaningful for the group members and relevant to the aim of the group. The activities need to be adaptable; it is important to have a plan B if it becomes obvious that the plans are not going to work. The group members may make choices about what they do and make decisions about the activities so become participative in the group leadership. Thought needs to be given about how much energy the group members put into each activity; sometimes it is important to introduce an activity which involves a lot of running around and swapping chairs when the energy level needs to be increased. You may want to move group members around so that they are sitting next to someone new. Possible activities include:

- Group discussion or debate
- Role play
- Games and quizzes
- Case studies
- Creative activities – art, music, drama
- Team building activities (Westergaard, 2009).

In early sessions I asked group members to work in pairs to discuss how their week had been. It was an effective way of helping the individuals who found it difficult to talk for a length of time to the whole group. Talking to one other person meant that they connected and shared similar experiences and feelings and they came to realise that their feelings were understood. After the exercise I asked each pair if there was anything that they wanted to share in the large group. There often was and more common experiences emerged. These common experiences would not have been raised if I had originally asked the group as a whole. I may have been met with silence.

Effective facilitation skills

The facilitation skills used in group work are very similar to those used in an individual counselling session; genuineness, empathy, being open, accepting and responsive. At the start of any group it is important to be positive and welcoming even if you are feeling unsure and anxious about the group yourself. After a 'how has the week been' activity I would usually summarise what has been discussed before moving on to the next activity. The difference in group facilitation is that you are summarising more than one person's experience. The important task here is to find connections in the shared experiences and emphasise learning points. For example: 'Last week we talked about how much we worry about other people judging us. Some people said that they ended up not meeting up with their friends at the weekend because they were so concerned about what people might say; and others said that sometimes they will find an excuse not to go to school because they are so anxious. So we learnt that anxiety makes us avoid situations which then affects our mood and makes us feel even less confident.' Another skill is to reflect back on the important issues that an individual has said and then ask the other group members what they think or if they have ever been in a similar situation. Facilitators and counsellors are encouraged not to give advice, it is more important that advice and opinion comes from group members.

Modelling behaviour

A group facilitator's behaviour will strengthen the norms and values of the group and may teach new behaviours. The relationship between the leader and co-leader is on view. Their discussions about group activities and decisions about the group and the individuals are on show. They are the parents of this group and group members see a different style of interaction than they are used to.

Scenario

I experienced a group member's feelings of anger at a perceived injustice. I remained seated and stayed calm which enabled the group member to vent her anger. I acknowledged the anger and the reasons for it, showed good active listening skills and did not retaliate or make excuses. Some of the other group members found the individual's anger frightening and wanted to step in and shout the person down to protect me. Some group members felt fear and wanted to run away. My co-leader reassured them that I was OK and did not need to be rescued and encouraged them to stay with the feelings and hear the person's anger. When the anger had subsided we discussed the views calmly. We also discussed my reaction and the perceptions of the co-leader and group members. The individual said that she was surprised that I had not got angry and slapped her or sent her out of the group. Other group members said that they had felt scared that the anger would turn into a fight. The learning that took place for the group members was a useful and new way of understanding and dealing with anger.

CO-LEADERSHIP

Not all groups have two co-leaders and it may be difficult and costly to arrange. In all of the groups I have run including psychotherapy or task and activity groups, I have found co-leadership invaluable. We often had a third person who was an apprentice group facilitator. Lindsay and Orton (2011) say co-facilitation is a useful way of learning by watching and participating gradually. The participants benefit from having different styles and more knowledge.

As in any relationship, co-leaders can have a healthy or unhealthy relationship. It is vital for the group members that the relationship is positive and communication open and honest. With co-leadership there is an opportunity for group members to manipulate and split the pair so good communication and supervision is essential. The pitfalls have been noted by Benson (2010) and he recommends against co-working. Lindsay and Orton disagree saying that provided time is taken to trust each other, the benefits outweigh the problems.

In groups that I facilitated in the past I would often have the role of explaining or leading the group in an activity. While I was explaining my co-leader would be checking the group members' reaction and non-verbal behaviour. She would step in and re-explain an activity, sometimes picking up a group member's confusion, or she would check the groups' understanding before moving on.

After the group finishes there is an opportunity for co-leaders to support one another, learn from one another and evaluate the group session, sharing the task of writing up the session and planning improvements for the next time the group runs.

NURTURING TRUST AND GROUP INCLUSION

Try to encourage the development of trust from the start of the group. Geldard and Geldard (2001) suggest the group leader models behaviour that indicates that they trust the group. Appropriate self-disclosure from the group leader can encourage the children to feel safe in disclosing themselves. It is sometimes difficult to assess what is appropriate self-disclosure. I very often stated at the start of anxiety management groups that I was anxious, that my heart was racing and I had butterflies in my stomach. This disclosure often surprised the group members and created a discussion about normal levels of anxiety. However it is not always appropriate to disclose on another occasion, and I decided not to disclose that someone close had died and that I was grieving for her. I think if I had shared this with the group I would be asking them for support. It was an unresolved problem for me and therefore it was inappropriate to share it with the group. Disclosing personal information that you have not resolved might mean that the group are concerned for your emotional safety and might make them feel that you are unable to keep them safe. Luxmoore (2008) also discusses disclosure and agrees that he has 'to model a degree of honesty'. He says things about himself that the group may not have expected: honest things and vulnerable things because he hopes that this will give permission for others to do the same.

The process of trust development is dynamic and can be changed by particular incidents. Group cohesion develops through acknowledgement of common elements, and it is a useful exercise before the first group ends to encourage clients to ask themselves, 'How can I get the most from this group?' The group leader can emphasise change and success by active participation and can concentrate on linking and connecting people by encouraging them to discuss their experiences. It is important not to force trust and to work directly using group members' behavioural and emotional expressions in a nurturing and accepting way.

COPING WITH CHALLENGES IN GROUPS

Activity

Think of a time when you have contributed to a problem within a group in the past. Do you have the same tendencies in groups and teams now?

When you are experiencing problems in groups it may be a good idea to ask:

- When is it a problem? – could it be uncomfortable, but productive?
- To whom is it a problem? – is it only the facilitator or to others?
- Why is the problem occurring? – is it caused by the activity, the environment, the leader's approach? Is the cause held within the group?

As a facilitator of groups I felt uncomfortable when dealing with problems and challenges. After a period of reflection many of the problems I have experienced in group work turned out to be opportunities rather than problems. Problems in groups could just be situations that we have not expected or planned for so they make us uncomfortable (Lindsay and Orton, 2011; Sharp and Cowie, 1998). However, it is important to deal with the events effectively as they could become bigger problems and make individuals' behaviours more entrenched and defensive. Group leaders need to be decisive and direct and use language that children can understand when dealing with problem behaviours (Geldard and Geldard, 2001).

Problems can occur in groups in relation to the environment in some cases, or may be problems to do with the leadership.

The environment

In the planning stage one of the early considerations is finding a suitable room to run the group. The size of the room, access to the room, lighting, temperature and the level of noise around the room are important factors. The room size, layout and furniture need to accommodate the type of group; so the room would be set out in a different way if it was an activity art group or a sharing supportive group. I have never run a group in a perfect location and have had to make do with sharing the group room with a pool table and dart board but it is a good idea to have the ideal room in mind before making a compromise. Geldard and Geldard (2001) suggest it should be safe and ensure that privacy and confidentiality are maintained. The group room should be free from auditory and visual distractions from outside (Geldard and Geldard, 2001). Some of the problems I have had to cope with are a large noisy lawn mower being used to cut the grass outside a room when I was trying to run a relaxation group, or an open plan art room where people who were not group members wandered into the group, and group rooms that were multi-functional so it was difficult to book them every week.

Leadership

The leader is sometimes the cause of problems in groups and even if they are not the cause may be scapegoated by the group members as a reaction to problems in the group. In groups with children and young people the group facilitators are likely to be the only adults and inevitably there will be either an actual or perceived power imbalance. Children are more likely to look to the adult for guidance or might see the leader as somebody whose authority needs to be challenged. Some of the problems are a result of poor planning by the leader. Finally the group leader may have personal problems that interfere with their facilitation skills during a group. Group leaders need to have the ability to cope with verbal attacks from group members without becoming defensive (Geldard and Geldard, 2001). Luxmoore (2008) is not surprised when young people who have self-esteem issues find being open in a group difficult. He describes his self-esteem group members stating that they all have ways of protecting themselves from shame. If this is the case then the worst strategy is to challenge them in the group.

STRATEGIES FOR DEALING WITH PROBLEMS

Silent individuals

The most obvious reason why someone is silent in the group is due to lack of confidence or anxiety. It is possible for the other members of a group to think that the silence is a threat to the group and the silent person to become a scapegoat. The group leader has the difficult responsibility to protect the individual whilst acknowledging the other group members feelings and allowing them to understand. The group leader needs to make sure that they continue to engage in eye contact with the person and not ignore the silent person. It is important to note that even though they are not contributing to the group they may be still engaging with the process. The group facilitator can engage the whole group in simple activities which encourage quiet members to participate in a non-threatening activity. Pair exercises are good because talking to one person and finding that you have something in common with them can break the ice and increase confidence. However it is possible that the group is not of any interest to them and the lack of engagement is due to boredom.

Strategies for dealing with a silent group member

- Accept the behaviour.
- Talk to the person on an individual basis.
- Encourage the person to communicate non-verbally.
- Direct the discussion within the group.
- Use pairs or smaller group work.
- Consider your own behaviour, in particular eye contact.

Dominating member

Just as anxiety is often the reason for silence in a group, anxiety can also be the reason for someone dominating the group. Dominating the group is a way of controlling the direction of the group away from issues that are difficult to handle. Some young people believe that unless they control people other people will control them (Luxmoore, 2008). When facilitating groups in substance misuse I noticed one group member would clown around and keep the group laughing; this process was a way of defending himself from the difficult subject matter and distracting the group from discussing painful subjects. Douglas (2000) notes that the person who sits opposite the group leader is often a potential challenge for the position of group leadership and he thinks that this may be because of the increased amount of eye contact the person would get in that position in the circle. Scrutiny from the leader gaze may make the person louder and more aggressive.

Strategies for dealing with a dominant member

- Talk to the person on an individual basis.
- Group leader sits next to the person thereby reducing eye contact and allowing light physical contact to discourage them from offering an opinion again.
- Direct and draw other members into discussion.
- Encourage the person to help other members to say more.
- Encourage group members to take responsibility for an aspect of the group.

Angry/distressed member

Anger is a way of coping when feeling exposed or threatened. Anger is a familiar bad feeling to some and feels safer than the feeling that is more appropriate for the situation. The biological explanation suggests that we are angry when we or a significant other are threatened or to meet our basic needs or to protect our space (Sharp and Cowie, 1998). I have noticed that feelings become confused when people are in a situation that is difficult to handle; anger is expressed instead of fear and people cry when they are furious. Luxmoore (2008) discusses a young group member's anger and wonders if creating conflict is a way for a young person to speed up the attachment process; ordinary attachment is too slow and uncertain and confrontation is more direct.

Strategies for dealing with an angry or distressed member

- Listen.
- Manage your own feelings.
- Consider the specific needs of the person concerned.
- Encourage constructive expression of emotion.
- Talk to the person on an individual basis.
- Attend to other group members.

Disruptive behaviour

There are many reasons for disruptive behaviour. The group member or members might feel coerced into the group and don't want to be there. They might feel uncomfortable with the subject matter or angry with a decision that is being made on their behalf. Young people who have a history of being disruptive in school might over-react to a perceived or actual criticism and revert to familiar reactions, trying to derail the group. They might simply be bored and want to increase the level of excitement or stimulation. They might be testing the leader out to see how they will react or be challenging other members of the group for the role of 'top dog'.

Strategies for dealing with disruptive behaviour

- Set clear expectations at the beginning of the group.
- Manage the behaviour through change of activity.
- Speak to the group member one to one.

Bizarre behaviour

In Tier 3 or 4 settings you may see children or young people with bizarre or unpredictable behaviour, probably due to their mental health condition.

Strategies for dealing with bizarre behaviour

- Attend to the degree of stimulation (quiet environment, simple activity).
- Attendance at some groups may not be appropriate.

Difficult situations affecting whole groups

Group work involves a high degree of unpredictability and this may be the factor that attracts you or puts you off facilitating groups. Over-controlling groups often leads to problems that affect the whole group. A group leader needs the ability to be flexible, to have a number of activities and plans in case the one that you had chosen is obviously not going to work. The most obvious reason for problems affecting whole groups is that the group aim is not a good match for the individual group members' needs.

A group in conflict

This occurs naturally in groups and is often the storming stage. Be aware of benefits of a 'storming' experience; it is important to discuss and be honest about the 'elephant in the room'. Group members need to be supported to experience healthy expression of feelings in a safe environment.

Strategies for the facilitator

- Use strategies previously discussed.
- Adapt the activity.
- Restructure the group if subgroups are emerging.
- Examine your own behaviour.

Silent group

Anxiety is one reason for a silent group; however I have facilitated many anxiety management groups and not many were silent. It is important to distinguish if the group is being silent or apathetic. If the group is silent it may be because they feel unsafe; if this is the case it is important to reflect on your leadership style and your preparation for the group. If group leaders appear unprepared it is natural for group members to doubt their ability to look after them. It may be that you have planned the group at the wrong developmental level and that the group members do not understand the concepts that you are putting across. If the group is apathetic they may be bored with the activity; the aims of the group may not be a good fit for their needs. The environment needs to be considered. Is the room too hot? Are you running the group straight after a large meal? Flexibility in group facilitation is imperative: always have a plan B and if the group are apathetic maybe an energetic fun activity is necessary.

Strategies to deal with the silent group

- Wait – see if the group responds. If you are a new leader your own anxiety may push you to intervene too quickly.
- Allow the silence; this can be hard but silence could be productive, it is thinking time.
- Examine your own response to the silence.
- Adapt the activity.

Strategies to deal with an apathetic group

- Examine own behaviour and leadership style.
- Change the activity.
- Employ trust building and cohesive exercises.

GROUP REFLECTION, EVALUATION AND SUPERVISION

Group workers may be tempted to think that the group is over when the group members leave. In a busy team supervision is often neglected; it is not seen as a priority and is often cancelled or rushed (Dwivedi, 1998). However it is extremely important to reflect and evaluate the session with co-workers. It is very useful for the development of facilitation skills and the support of the facilitators to have regular supervision from a person outside the group. Evaluation should be seen as an integral part of the group process (Westergaard, 2009); documenting the evaluation is also important. Workers may discuss how the session could be improved next time it runs and any changes that may need to occur for the following session. Each co-worker will have a slightly different perspective of what has occurred in the session. Co-workers will have noticed different non-verbal behaviours communicated by participants in the group. It is important for co-workers to share their feelings and observations (Dwivedi, 1998).

CONCLUSION

Group work with children and young people can take more organisation and is often more anxiety provoking than individual work with children and young people but the benefits can be far reaching. Participants find opportunities to connect with other young people and test out new ways of relating to each other within a safe and supportive environment.

REFERENCES

Benson, J.F. (2010) *Working Creatively with Groups*, 3rd edn. London: Routledge.

Burnard, P. (1990) *Learning Human Skills: An Experiential Guide for Nurses*. Oxford: Butterworth Heinemann.

Campion, J. (1991) *Counselling Children*. London: Whiting and Birch.

Cole, M.B. (2005) *Group Dynamics in Occupational Therapy*. Thorofare, NJ: Slack Inc.

Cooper, P. (1999) *Understanding and Supporting Children with Emotional and Behavioural Difficulties* London: Jessica Kingsley.

Cooper, P. and Tiknaz, Y. (2007) *Nurture Groups in School and at Home: Connecting with Children with Social, Emotional and Behavioural Difficulties*. London: Jessica Kingsley.

Doel, M. (2007) *Using Groupwork*. London: Routledge.

Douglas, T. (2000) *Basic Groupwork*. London: Routledge.

Drost, J. and Bayley, S. (2001) *Therapeutic Groupwork with Children*. Milton Keynes: Speechmark Publishing.

Dwivedi, K.N. (1998) *Group Work with Children and Adolescents*, 3rd edn. London: Jessica Kingsley.

Geldard, K. and Geldard, D. (2001) *Working with Children in Groups: A Handbook for Counsellors, Educators and Community Workers*. Basingstoke: Palgrave.

Geldard, K. and Geldard, D. (2008) *Counselling Children : A Practical Introduction*, 3rd edn. London: Sage.

Hamori, E. and Hodi, A. (1996) Reflection of Family Transference in Group Psychotherapy for Preadolescents. *Group Analysis*, 29 (1): 43–54.

Lewin, K., Lippit, R. and White, R.K. (1939) Patterns of Aggressive Behavior in Experimentally Created 'Social Climates'. *Journal of Social Psychology*, 10: 271–301.

Lindsay, T. and Orton, S. (2011) *Groupwork Practice in Social Work*, 2nd edn. Exeter: Learning Matters.

Lloyd, C., Waghorn, G., Williams, P., Harris, M. and Capra, C. (2008) Early Psychosis: Treatment Issues and the Role of Occupational Therapy. *British Journal of Occupational Therapy*, 71 (7): 97–304

Luxmoore, N. (2008) *Feeling Like Crap: Young People and the Meaning of Self-esteem*. London: Jessica Kingsley.

McDermott, F. (2002) *Inside Groupwork*. Sydney: Allen and Unwin.

Preston-Shoot, M. (2007) *Effective Groupwork*. Basingstoke: Palgrave Macmillan.

Prever, M. (2011) *Counselling and Supporting Children and Young People: A Person-centred Approach*. London: Sage.

Rose, S.R. (1998) *Group Work with Children and Adolescents: Prevention and Intervention in School and Community Systems*. London: Sage.

Sharp, S. and Cowie, H. (1998) *Counselling and Supporting Children in Distress*. London: Sage.

Tuckman, B.W. (1965) Developmental Sequence in Small Groups. *Psychological Bulletin*, 63 (6): 384–99.

Westergaard, J. (2009) *Effective Group Work with Young People Berkshire*. Maidenhead: Open University Press.

8

VALUES, ATTITUDES, BELIEFS AND INEQUALITIES WHEN WORKING WITH CHILDREN, YOUNG PEOPLE AND THEIR FAMILIES

ERICA PAVORD, BRIONY WILLIAMS AND MADDIE BURTON

Overview

- Definition of terms
- How values, beliefs and attitudes are formed
- Equality, inequality and discrimination
- How discrimination impacts on children, young people and their families
- How to practise in an anti-discriminatory way
- Anti-discriminatory legislation and strategies

INTRODUCTION

This chapter aims to explore and reflect on values, attitudes, beliefs, prejudices and inequalities in relation to working with children, young people and their families. It is vital to acknowledge at the outset that children, regardless of anything else, are often discriminated against because they are children, and their ideas, rights and experiences are often considered less important or relevant than those of the adults in their lives.

Britain in the 21st century is a culturally rich and diverse society and services have to respond to the needs of this society through practices which both value the diversity and address the linguistic and cultural needs of the population. Social policy promotes agendas which are anti-discriminatory and inclusive and which tackle the uncomfortable truth of institutional racism.

> Meeting the mental health needs of ethnic minority children at every level of service delivery challenges us all to consider the culture and style of our service organisations.
> (Brinley Harper and Dwivedi, 2004: 234)

It is not only the needs of ethnic minorities but all minorities that we must take into account. The Equality Act 2010 identifies the following protected characteristics which ensure that people with these characteristics are protected from discrimination:

- Age
- Disability
- Gender reassignment
- Marriage and civil partnership
- Pregnancy and maternity
- Race
- Religion or belief
- Sex
- Sexual orientation.

In all services and organisations working with children, young people and their families, practitioners need to demonstrate non-judgemental attitudes and to promote anti-discriminatory practice. This chapter creates an opportunity for you to explore the causes and impact of prejudice, discrimination and inequality in various settings. It will encourage you to identify strategies which combat and promote anti-discriminatory practice. You will be asked to reflect on your own values, attitudes and beliefs and to gain greater awareness of how they can impact on your work. It provides a space for consideration and reflection of your perspectives on difference and diversity.

DEFINING TERMS

Beliefs, values and attitudes

Beliefs, values and attitudes are linked:

- *Beliefs* are the assumptions we make about ourselves, others and the world we live in. Some beliefs are held by most cultures in the world, such as 'taking another human life is wrong', but some are specific to particular groups of people or to individuals and are often dependent on environment and experiences. A person who has lived through a war or through natural disaster might have a belief that the world is a dangerous place. Those who choose to work with children and young people might share the belief that adults have a duty to care for and protect children.
- A *value* is usually formed by a particular belief and is something that is important or worth something to us. Values can have financial, emotional, personal or professional worth and can be shared by many or held by just one person. We may see value in physical objects because of their financial value or their beauty or the emotional attachment we have to them. We might value ways of being like kindness, assertiveness, friendliness. In the context of working ethically with children, young people and their families, our personal and professional values guide us in our decision making, actions and interactions with others. Values are hard to quantify, standardise or evidence but their impact is fundamental (Cuthbert and Quallington, 2008). Some of the values that are particularly important in working in child and adolescent mental health settings are:

  - Compassion
  - Empathy
  - Sincerity
  - Trustworthiness
  - Integrity
  - Respectfulness (Beauchamp and Childress, 2001).

- An *attitude* is the way a person expresses or applies their beliefs and values, and is expressed through words and behaviour. Attitudes are the established ways of responding to people and situations that we have learned, based on the beliefs, values and assumptions we hold. If we have a belief that children must be cared for and protected from harm and we value compassion and empathy, our attitude will be one of kindness and thoughtfulness, listening to the young people we work with and valuing their opinions.

PERSONAL AND PROFESSIONAL VALUES

Values can be observed on three different but interrelated levels:

- On an individual level and the extent to which we value our moral integrity and are true to ourselves.

- In our interactions with others and how we communicate with the people around us.
- On a societal level and how we value community and the wider society.

Our personal values have an impact on how we value our interactions with others and with society and our workplace and vice versa. It is often the case that people who choose to work with children and young people have similar core values and these are reflected in the professional values laid out in the set of standards or code of conduct of a particular professional body (Cuthbert and Quallington, 2008). Sometimes these values clash and we have to decide where to position ourselves in relation to what society or our workplace demands. For example a teacher might value the individuality of his pupils and place no particular personal value on school uniform but the school has a strict uniform policy and he has to give detentions to pupils who won't adhere to the policy. A nurse who believes in no sex before marriage might be working with young girls who are sexually active and want advice on contraception. In situations like these and many others it is important that we find a balance between holding onto our personal values whilst respecting the professional values we work within.

Activity

Make a list of your core values, things you are not willing to compromise over?
Now put this list in order of importance to you.
Now try and say why each one is important.
I believe.........................because.....................
e.g. I believe that it is wrong to intentionally harm another person because you should treat others the way you would want to be treated yourself.

HOW BELIEFS, VALUES AND ATTITUDES ARE FORMED

We all live by some personal value base and are not always aware of where this value base comes from. Our values may have been passed down from parents, grandparents or significant others when we were growing up. Or values may become conscious and are reinforced and given clarity by important, meaningful, critical incidents in our lives. Sometimes these incidents are in the work setting when we see or are involved in a situation which makes us uncomfortable and our feelings of discomfort tell us that our values are being challenged.

The development of beliefs and values starts in childhood and continues throughout our lives. We begin to acquire them from our parents and care givers from early childhood and these are added to by cultural norms in education and play. Words like 'be kind', 'don't snatch', 'wait your turn', are heard so many times that they are assimilated into our moral make-up. Our development of morals and values are influenced by many factors as we grow up: parents, siblings, teachers, friends, peer groups, media, culture, religion, political ideologies. Some have become the basic moral foundations of right and wrong, good and bad, but some are subjective and dependent on our individual experience. Some values can be transitory and fleeting, influenced by friends or fashion and some are deep rooted and difficult to shift. A person who has grown up with a core belief that the world is a dangerous place might value cautiousness. Their attitude is likely to be one of mistrust and fearfulness. In time, if the belief is challenged and they start to experience new things which help them to grow in confidence they might start to change their values, but if they are continually reinforced this is less likely.

Activity

I was brought up in a high-achieving family that valued hard work, academic and professional success. It was expected that I and my siblings would go to university and get good, well-paid jobs. In my teens and twenties I was quite judgemental about people who didn't share this value and I was certainly self-critical when I felt that I wasn't achieving enough. However, over the years my work has meant that I have challenged this belief time and time again. I have worked with individuals and families who have had very different experiences to my own and who don't share my values and this has led me to change my beliefs, particularly in relation to other people. If I were still judgemental about this I would not be working ethically, I would be judging people according to my own values and beliefs and this would have a detrimental effect on my ability to form a therapeutic relationship with my clients.

What values have you acquired or rejected as you've grown up?

THE CAUSES AND IMPACT OF STEREOTYPING, PREJUDICE, INEQUALITY AND DISCRIMINATION

When people's beliefs and values are based on faulty and inflexible generalisations they can result in stereotyping and prejudice and this can lead to discrimination (Allport, 1954). In addressing issues of equality and discrimination it is important to understand what is meant by the terms used.

Stereotype

When we assume that people of shared physical, religious, cultural or other characteristics have certain behavioural attributes, this is called a stereotype. It is very easy to stereotype and it often goes unchallenged. We frequently hear phrases like 'boys don't like talking about their feelings' or 'girls are so emotional' and many would agree with these statements based on their experience of working with young people but the danger is that by not questioning stereotypes, we are less likely to relate to each person as an individual. Stereotypes are often offensive in that they are reductive and generalised and often single out one characteristic which is forced on individuals or groups of people as if they are indistinguishable from each other. We need to remember that there is never a single story about a person or a group of people. Stereotypes are not necessarily wrong because they are untrue but because they are incomplete, they make one story become the only story (Adiche, 2009). Understanding individuals and their cultural context is a far more positive approach than generalising according to stereotyped ideas.

Prejudice

> A prejudice is an opinion or judgement formed without considering the relevant facts; a strongly held attitude. (Webb and Tossell, 1999: 14)

Prejudice is often based on stereotypes and takes stereotyping a step further. The word is usually associated with negative connotations and quite often it involves negative feelings such as mistrust, anger, fear and sometimes hatred. Prejudice can be directed at individuals or groups and is justified by those holding the prejudice because they have attributed stereotypical traits to those who are the focus of the prejudice; 'teenage mothers are irresponsible scroungers' or 'young black men are violent and angry'.

According to Allport (1954), a prejudice may involve a number of processes:

Cognitive: a false belief that one person or group is superior to another.

Emotional: the belief leads to an emotional response; a feeling, usually negative, towards another person or group.

Discriminatory action: the feeling or belief is acted on in a number of different ways; by ignoring the other person or group, saying unpleasant things about them or deliberately taking some kind of unfair action against them.

As human beings it is almost impossible not to hold some prejudices and it is important that we are accepting of this, reflect on the impact of our prejudice on the people we come into contact with and ensure that our prejudices do not lead to discriminatory actions. It is also important to reflect on where our prejudices come from and be understanding of how the children, young people and families we work with formed theirs. For example a young woman who has been in and out of care and has had a long line of social workers and foster carers making decisions for her might well hold a strong prejudice against social services and workers which then affects the way that she deals with authority figures in her life.

Prejudices are sometimes difficult to identify because they can be deeply rooted in our core beliefs. A worker in children's services might have a firmly held prejudice against parents who abuse drugs and alcohol and not question that prejudice because her experience has shown her that many children suffer when living with drug and alcohol abuse. However, it is important to recognise that this is a prejudice and inevitably affects the way that the worker communicates with parents and children who are affected. It is easy to make assumptions about people when we hold onto prejudice and to stop seeing them as individuals.

Different kinds of prejudice

- *Racism:* believing that skin colour, ethnicity or culture makes certain people inferior.
- *Classism:* believing that certain economic classes are superior.
- *Sexism:* believing that sex and gender determine status.
- *Lookism:* believing that appearance and looks determine status.
- *Homophobia/heterosexism:* believing that sexual or gender orientation makes one group inferior.
- *Ableism:* believing that physical and/or mental ability makes one group superior.
- *Ageism:* believing that age determines status.

Discrimination

Discrimination can be defined in different ways. At its most basic level discrimination is simply a matter of identifying differences and this can be positive and negative. In certain situations it is important to discriminate between certain things or people in order to ensure fairness. A teacher of a class of children with differing abilities must discriminate between different pupils to ensure that each has an equal opportunity to achieve. Negative discrimination however is very different as it involves identifying difference by making negative assumptions about a person or a group of people.

When negative discrimination occurs the resulting experience is usually one of oppression. Thompson (2006: 40) describes discrimination as:

> Inhuman or degrading treatment of individuals or groups; hardship and injustice brought about by the dominance of one group over another; the negative and demeaning exercise of power. It often involves disregarding the rights of an individual or group and is thus a denial of citizenship.

Personal, cultural, structural analysis (PCS)

To help us to understand discrimination and the oppression that arises from it, it is useful to recognise that it operates at three different, interrelated levels: personal, cultural and structural (Thompson, 2011).

The *personal* is concerned with our own thoughts feelings and actions and manifests itself as prejudice. We make judgements about people or groups of people and discriminate based on our own beliefs and values. It is purely related to individual actions and you are likely to come into contact with this in practice. Sometimes people are overtly discriminatory, like a teacher who won't allow girls on the school football team. Sometimes people are unaware of their prejudice, like a professional who assumes that a black family is uneducated because they live in a poor area. When challenged, this professional might be deeply offended that they are accused of being prejudiced but their assumption reveals a level of underlying racism. Discrimination that occurs at a personal level is inextricably linked to an individual's context and experience, which means that it is embedded in the cultural level of discrimination.

The *cultural* is concerned with the way of life of a group of people and the shared patterns of thinking, feeling and behaving. Discrimination occurs when a group of

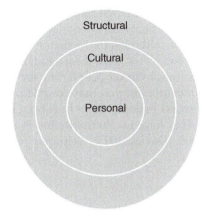

Figure 8.1 PCS Analysis, Adapted from Thompson (2011)

people create an 'us and them' situation dependent on the perceived superiority of one group over another. Often we can become so immersed in the shared assumptions and values that we don't even notice they are there or question the evidence. We only have to look at the media to see how embedded certain assumptions have become. Headlines in national newspapers fuel common cultural myths and prejudices:

IT'S NOT RACIST TO STATE THAT GYPSY CAMPS FREQUENTLY CAUSE AN INCREASE IN CRIME AND MESS – IT IS A STATEMENT OF FACT. (*Daily Mail*, Phibbs, 2009)

THESE KIDS WILL NICK ANYTHING FOR DRUGS. (*Daily Telegraph*, Savill, 2002)

Just as the personal level of discrimination in PCS analysis must be understood within the wider context of culture, so must the cultural level be seen through the wider lens of society as a whole.

The *structural* is concerned with the social, political and economic ideas that underpin policy. Social factors are related to class, ethnicity, gender and other social divisions. Political factors involve the distribution of power both formally and informally. Economic factors are concerned with the distribution of wealth and other material resources. By thinking about the personal and cultural levels of discrimination within the wider structural context we see how interrelated they are. To challenge racism or sexism on a purely personal or cultural level we are ignoring the reality that at a structural level power is traditionally in the hands of white men. 'Sexist assumptions and cultural patterns do not arise as a matter of coincidence – they are explained by reference to the need to protect vested interests, in this case, to maintain men in positions of power and privilege' (Thompson, 2011: 30). The analysis of discrimination at a structural level shows how it is 'sewn into the fabric of society' through institutions that support both cultural norms and personal beliefs. Some institutions such as sections of the media, religion and the government can reinforce these beliefs, giving them a sense of permanence and acceptability. This, until the Marriage (Same Sex Couples) Act 2013, was clearly illustrated in the way that homophobic attitudes, both personal and cultural, were underpinned by inequalities in the church and state around the rights of same sex couples to get married. Discrimination can also occur indirectly in perhaps less obvious ways. It is not necessarily about setting out to discriminate but that actions result in discrimination, although the 'perpetrator' may not be aware of this at the time. Indirect discrimination takes place throughout all levels of society from government, organisations, institutions to the people who are part of them. A recent local example of indirect discrimination (or you may consider it is direct) is a new sloping footpath built to access a sports building. Steps have been built in so wheelchair users cannot use the new path. They have no alternative but to use the old path, which is a much longer, circuitous route (Davies, 2013). Below are two case studies to consider.

Activity

Have a look at the following scenario and consider:

- *Do you think an appropriate decision was made?*
- *If you agree or disagree, what do you think are the corresponding implications?*

Saira is 14 and a daughter to South Asian parents. She was born in the UK although her parents were not. When Saira was 11 she was diagnosed with early onset schizophrenia. Following that diagnosis she has been in and out of Tier 4 CAMHS in-patient units. Recently she was sectioned; she is currently under Section 3 of the Mental Health Act 1983, amended 2007. (This is a Section for 'treatment' and is of six months' duration.)

Sunday evening is visiting time on the ward for the parents and families of the young people. Saira's parents and her siblings arrive to spend the evening with her. They have brought some food, prepared at home, which they plan to share with Saira.

A nurse on duty tells Saira she cannot have the food her parents have brought in. The nurse tells Saira and the family that she did not eat the ward meal offered earlier that evening, which means she cannot have anything to eat now with her family.

Saira and her family are quite upset about this but they are generally uncomplaining and accept the decision of the nurse without a fuss.

Response

The above scenario contains many issues but is a useful example of indirect discrimination. The nurse may not have set out to treat Saira differently but her actions mean that Saira is being treated differently and potentially is being discriminated against. Saira's culture would include bringing in food from home and sharing with a family member who was hospitalised as Saira is. Other children on the ward might go out with their families to a café in the local town to share a meal together; what is the difference when Saira and her family chose to do this on the ward? Parents of ethnic minority children can often feel intimidated by majority cultures and in this scenario a dominant 'western' culture with regard to psychiatry. They are often less likely to challenge 'treatment' as Saira's family were.

It also means that potentially Saira will not have eaten for a long time given she has missed the ward meal (which does have cultural options for Saira) and is not having any food from home. Her next meal would be the next day at breakfast.

You can probably consider several other issues and implications in addition to the above.

Activity

Have a look at the following case and consider whether the school arrived at the right decision and is indirect discrimination taking place?

John is 7. He has a diagnosis of ADHD. The school John attends is concerned about his safety at playtime. They consider his lack of impulse control means he is likely to run off out of the school and place himself at obvious risk.

The school takes the decision to instruct mum to dress John in an alternative colour to the standard school uniform. All the other pupils wear a blue sweatshirt. They ask mum to dress John in a red top. This is so he will be seen easily amongst the other school children and therefore be immediately identified. Mum objects to this.

Response

John has a diagnosis of ADHD, which is a recognised disability and therefore he is protected in law by the Equality Act 2010. Asking him to wear different clothing as a consequence of his ADHD is unfairly and illegally treating him differently to the other children. School may have thought of this idea with every good intention in terms of John's safety. However not taking other safety measures, such as keeping the school gate closed, is another aspect of indirect discrimination. Children with impulse control are less likely to run out of the gate; in order to manage John he is being treated differently by being asked to wear different clothing. Instead, why don't they just shut the gate for everyone's safety?

Asking individuals to wear something different to further identify their individual 'difference' offers unpleasant reminders in history in relation to the persecution of the Jews in the Second World War. Individuals were forced to be identified with symbols and made to wear the Star of David to identify them outwardly as different.

As with the previous case you can probably consider several other issues and implications in addition to the above.

Equality

The concept of equality, like discrimination, can be defined on different levels. The literal meaning of equality is 'sameness' but it is more complex than this, particularly in a moral and legal sense. If we were to practise equality in its literal sense we would be treating everyone the same, which only reinforces injustice. In its moral and legal sense, equality refers to 'equal fairness', making sure that individuals or groups are treated fairly and have equality of opportunity (Thompson, 2011). So, applying the principles of equality in practical terms within child and adolescent mental health, all children and young people should have equal access to services regardless of their cultural and ethnic background, skin colour, religion, ability, gender and sexual orientation. Failure to respect another's right to equality puts them at a disadvantage (Cuthbert and Quallington, 2008). This can happen unintentionally because of a practitioner's lack of experience or effectiveness; it is easy to see why the needs of one child whose parents are more demanding are prioritised over the needs of another who has no one in their corner or who waits patiently for their turn. Situations like this are common and although they occur without malice or intention to discriminate, they should be guarded against. 'Equality can be understood as an absence of (unfair) discrimination, a situation where people are not treated unfairly simply because they are different in some way' (Thompson, 2011: 7).

Inequality

The opposite of equality is inequality and it describes the gap that exists between people or groups. It often refers to the gap in income and resources between rich and poor, but inequalities in people's economic positions are also related to their characteristics – whether they are men or women, their ages, ethnic backgrounds and so on (Hills et al., 2010). Inequality acts as a barrier to individuals reaching their potential and discovering their talents; it can also stifle emotional wellbeing and impact negatively on mental health. Research has found that:

> ... almost all problems which are more common at the bottom of the social ladder are more common in more unequal societies. (Wilkinson and Pickett, 2009: 18)

Despite many efforts to tackle inequality, we live in an unequal society. A report published in January 2010 (Hills et al., 2010) pointed out that inequality in Britain had increased over the last 10 years with the household wealth of the top 10% standing at over 100 times higher than that of the poorest 10%. Inevitably economic inequality affects the most vulnerable, and those with the least power in an unequal society are often the greatest victims. Children and young people are usually the most vulnerable in society and have the least power, so they are inevitably the most affected by inequality.

Culture

It is useful to define the word culture here as it is a concept that is integral to discussions around values, attitudes and beliefs and often understood as applying to ethnicity.

There are many definitions of 'culture' and it is not a value-free concept (Dogra, 2007). As professionals we need to engage actively with the concept of culture, cultural identity or belonging to a cultural group as it is too simplistic to define culture by assigning particular characteristics like ethnicity. Dogra (2007) cites the Association of American Medical Colleges to provide a useful definition:

> Culture is defined by each person in relationship to the group or groups with whom he or she identifies. An individual's cultural identity may be based on heritage as well as individual circumstances and personal choice. Cultural identity may be affected by factors such as race, ethnicity, age, language, country of origin, acculturation, sexual orientation, gender, socioeconomic status, religious/spiritual beliefs, physical abilities, occupation, among others. These factors may impact on behaviours such as communication styles, diet preferences, health beliefs, family roles, lifestyle, rituals and decision making processes. All of these beliefs and practices, in turn can influence how patients and health care professionals perceive health and illness, and how they interact with one another. (Association of American Medical Colleges, 1999: 25)

Diversity

Traditional equal opportunities policy and practice focus on tackling discriminatory practice. A more positive reframing of issues of equality is to celebrate difference and capitalise on the richness of background, culture and experience that exists in our society. Valuing diversity is a means of promoting equality and building on positives rather than attempting to reduce negatives (Thompson, 2011: 11). It is a forward looking perspective that sees difference and variety as an asset, something valuable and positive. Walker (1994) proposed a 'Valuing Differences' model which is based on the following principles:

- People work best when they feel valued.
- People feel most valued when they believe that their individual and group differences have been taken into account.
- The ability to learn from people regarded as different is the key to becoming fully empowered.
- When people feel valued and empowered, they are able to build relationships in which they work together interdependently and synergistically (Walker, 1994: 212).

Activity

Think about your past and current experience: Identify times when diversity has been celebrated and reflect on the impact that has had on you.

THE IMPACT OF PERSONAL AND CULTURAL VALUES AND PREJUDICES IN OUR WORK

In the majority of settings where professionals work with children, young people and their families there are policies and practices in place to ensure that equality is promoted and discrimination is avoided. This will be looked at in more detail later in the chapter, so the focus here will be on an individual level and will explore how our own beliefs, values, attitudes and prejudices can impact on the people we work with. Reflecting on our practice and how our values impact on our interactions with others is essential.

Activity

Reflect on a time when you know that your personal beliefs and values have clashed with those of another person (particularly in your helping/professional role). Use the Gibbs cycle of reflection (Jasper, 1988) in Chapter 6 to help you to think about how this incident might have impacted on you, the other person and the relationship.

In order to work effectively and in a culturally sensitive way we must take into account our own values, attitudes and beliefs and the influence of current events and how they affect our day-to-day functioning. It is essential to be open and honest about our prejudices and how they affect our interactions. In any situation, issues around diversity inevitably have an impact even when we are not aware of it. Burnham et al. (2008) developed the following acronym which he called the Social GRRAACCEESS to assist professionals working therapeutically with families, reminding them to be mindful of the multitude of issues surrounding diversity that can affect the relationship.

Gender

Race

Religion

Age

Ability

Class

Culture

Ethnicity

Education

Sexuality

Spirituality

The issues that arise in therapeutic relationships with children, adolescents and their families might vary between being:

... visible and voiced; visible and unvoiced; invisible and voiced; and invisible and unvoiced, and all movements in between. (Burnham et al., 2008: 529).

Figure 8.2 gives examples of situations where visible and invisible differences might impact on the interaction between two people.

When differences are spoken about openly there is less potential for misunderstandings which result from stereotyping. This is not to say that we should always be open about our differences as it is sometimes more appropriate for them to remain unvoiced and invisible. In these cases it is important to remain curious about a child or young person's context or the impact of our own context rather than assuming that we are the same. Although certain issues may be invisible and unvoiced with the client, they shouldn't be when we reflect on our practice. Cecchin (1987), one of the founders of the Milan systemic therapy school, reflected that it is only when we are able to recognise our own attitudes and presumptions that we can begin to work ethically with clients. Our prejudices can be useful to us in that they encourage us to reflect on our own beliefs and how they interact with the beliefs of the people we are working with. We need to question the invisible as well as the visible difference as the obvious dissimilarity is easier to take into account than the assumed equality (Halson, 2005).

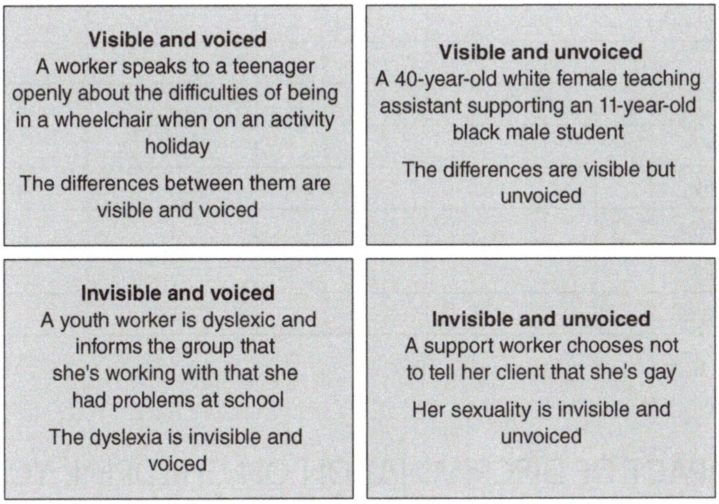

Visible and voiced A worker speaks to a teenager openly about the difficulties of being in a wheelchair when on an activity holiday The differences between them are visible and voiced	**Visible and unvoiced** A 40-year-old white female teaching assistant supporting an 11-year-old black male student The differences are visible but unvoiced
Invisible and voiced A youth worker is dyslexic and informs the group that she's working with that she had problems at school The dyslexia is invisible and voiced	**Invisible and unvoiced** A support worker chooses not to tell her client that she's gay Her sexuality is invisible and unvoiced

Figure 8.2 Visible and invisible, voiced and unvoiced differences

Activity

Read the following example and discuss the issues which might come up in the work this woman is doing with the boy and his foster family.

> A 45-year-old white, middle-class family support worker, educated to Master's level with a previous background in teaching. She has a mixed race child who has no contact with her father. She is married to a white man and they have a son. The support worker is working with a 14-year-old boy and the foster family he has been living with for five years. The boy is mixed race, his birth mother, who is a drug user, is white and she has never discussed his father with him. The boy's foster family are white and they are practising Christians. The boy has been referred because of his angry outbursts at home and in school and his hostility towards his foster parents. The support worker has all this information on referral. Using the form in Figure 8.3, reflect on the various visible and invisible, voiced and unvoiced issues that might come up in the relationship between the support worker and this family.

This is a useful activity to practice with a colleague as it creates opportunity for narrative or story and increases self-awareness and reflexivity.

Social GRRAACCEESS	Visible	Invisible	Voiced	Unvoiced
Gender				
Race				
Religion				
Age				
Ability				
Class				
Culture				
Ethnicity				
Education				
Sexuality				
Spirituality				

Figure 8.3

THE IMPACT OF DISCRIMINATION ON CHILDREN, YOUNG PEOPLE AND THEIR FAMILIES

In every interaction with young people and their families, whatever their background, we must consider the impact of our own values. If we are not alert to the way that our values, attitudes and beliefs impact on the young people we work with we risk alienating them and their families and increasing the risk to their mental health. There are particular groups of people who are more vulnerable to discrimination than others and these are referred to in the Equality Act 2010. This chapter cannot address all vulnerable groups so it will focus on the impact discrimination can have on ethnic minorities and people with disabilities. Brinley Harper and Dwivedi (2004) point out that the uptake of child and adolescent mental health services by ethnic minorities is notoriously poor and if they are accessed, tend to be inappropriate or alienating because of a lack of understanding and cultural sensitivity. The same might be said of the experiences of children with physical or learning disabilities whose mental health needs are overlooked in the efforts to address their physical and learning needs.

ETHNICITY

Ethnicity refers to the shared cultural traits and shared group history that certain groups of people have. It is a more useful and meaningful term to describe groups of people rather than 'Race', which is problematic in that it refers to specific biological traits like skin colour and assumes that we can separate out groups of people according to the colour of their skin or facial features. Whereas we are all humans, members of one 'human race'. Identity is based on a complexity of factors including and beyond physical characteristics. These lines are often blurred between an individual's personal identity, and how they are seen by others. This is why it is so important for us to avoid assumptions based on physical appearance and to spend time getting to know and understand the individual and what is important to them and their sense of identity.

In general, people from black and ethnic minority groups living in the UK are:

- More likely to be diagnosed with mental health problems;
- More likely to be diagnosed and admitted to hospital;
- More likely to experience a poor outcome from treatment;
- More likely to disengage from mainstream mental health services;
- More likely to be socially excluded (Mental Health Foundation, 2013).

> People from ethnic minorities have to overcome 'double discrimination' (a co-incidence of mental illness and minority status) when they seek help for treatment of mental illness for themselves or their children. It is no wonder that their underuse of services is an almost universal reality. (Banhatti and Bhate, 2002: 82)

The emotional wellbeing and mental health of black and ethnic minority children and young people is negatively impacted by racism and discrimination in some of the following ways:

- The development of an inferiority complex, low self-esteem and internalised racism so that children believe that they are not as good as or valued as their white peers.
- Problems of assimilation so that children and young people relate more to the majority culture and less to their own.
- Problems of separation where children and young people feel isolated and marginalised from the majority culture and identify exclusively with their own culture.
- Issues of biculturalism where children and young people have multiple identities due to living within a number of cultures and not having one stable identity (Coleman, 2011).

The impact of prejudice and cultural insensitivity on children and young people from ethnic minorities accessing mental health services are explored by Brinley Harper and Dwivedi (2004). They identify particular barriers to black and ethnic minority families accessing services.

Help seeking behaviour and stigmatisation

People from ethnic minority backgrounds are also less likely than white British to seek treatment for mental illness so it is inevitable that they are less likely to seek support for the emotional and mental health needs of their children.

Mistrust

The impact of historical racism, segregation and discrimination has meant that some ethnic minority families are fearful of accessing services because of the threat of hostile and untrustworthy professionals. Ethnic minorities who are experiencing mental health issues may be nervous about going to seek support from services because of the possibility of being incorrectly diagnosed or encountering institutional racism (Salway et al., 2013). If they continue to be disengaged from support and treatment, mental health problems can worsen, leading to crisis such as harm to self or others.

The use of jargon, patterns of speech and other traditional communication methods can be alienating and seen as the domain of majority culture professionals. A logical solution to this would be for there to be more professionals from a black and ethnic minority background who have some insight and understanding of the cultural and linguistic needs of ethnic minority children and their families.

Professional bias

Psychiatry in the UK is based on a western understanding of mental illness that there is something 'wrong' with a person's make-up that must be put right, usually using medication to correct a chemical imbalance in the brain. However, other cultures may see mental illness in terms of the mental and spiritual experience of a person.

Because many services do not engage with people in a holistic way, some people from black and minority ethnic communities (or BME) may be discouraged from seeking help, or find that their mental health problems are not recognised when they do.

In the mental health field, diagnosis relies heavily on behavioural signs rather than physical symptoms. White, western professionals in CAMHS settings are susceptible to misinterpreting certain behaviours because of an often unconscious cultural bias which results in either over- or under-diagnosing mental illness. Children, adolescents and their families are at risk of being given inappropriate advice or treatment that is based on a Eurocentric belief system at odds with their own:

> [The] Western view emphasises independence, self sufficiency, assertiveness, competition and mastery of the environment. Self fulfilment is dependent on doing … Verbal and direct communicational modes are valued. The non Western-European view, particularly the Oriental view, emphasises interdependence and harmony and co-operation in relationships. Self fulfilment is dependent on being. Non-verbal, indirect communication through the use of shared symbols is traditionally valued as a higher communication mode. (Lau, 1994: 7).

Cultural differences such as these give rise to misunderstanding. For example, professionals assume that independence from the family is a cultural norm for older adolescents and interpret obedience and respect as low self-esteem and lack of assertiveness. For bicultural young people from ethnic minorities who are torn between the western culture of their schools and peers and the culture of their families, it is important that professionals avoid colluding with them against their families and their cultural beliefs. It is all too common for professionals to be critical of restrictive parents without thinking about their cultural, religious and community beliefs. There is a tendency to stereotype and assume knowledge of a particular culture without taking into account the multiple layers of meaning that exist in any interaction between professionals and children, young people and their families.

Activity

Reflect or discuss with a partner what the cultural issues are in the following situation (assuming that there are no safeguarding issues):
   The male nurse of a Pakistani Muslim girl wants to speak with her alone but has so far only been able to speak to her father who does not want her to speak.

Language and the use of interpreters

Access to services is often inhibited by language barriers, particularly in migrant families, refugees and asylum seekers. One of the main features of good communication in CAMHS is the relationship between the young person and the professional and the rapport and trust that is built up between them. Most good relationships are reliant on good interpersonal communication and this is immediately hindered by language barriers. Sometimes it will be necessary to use an interpreter with a young person or family who does not speak English. Interpreting is essential if non-English speakers are to gain access to mental health services, and not offering this service could be seen as discriminatory (Smith, 2008). The job of the interpreter is complex as they need to know two languages well and be able to interpret both the spoken word and the tone and pace of both parties. They act as interpreters, not only of language, but also of meaning and cultural information. It is very hard to find interpreters who can work therapeutically alongside the professional and sometimes it will be necessary to use family members or friends or people with little knowledge of mental health issues, and so breakdown in communication still occurs. There are also issues of confidentiality, secrecy and shame so families who need an interpreter have to trust that not only the professional, but that the interpreter will adhere to confidentiality and ethical guidelines.

DISABILITY

Children and young people who are disabled are doubly challenged: first, their disability brings with it certain restrictions which make it more difficult for them to have the same opportunities as their peers; second, they have to deal with the challenges of other people's often patronising attitudes to their disability:

> It is the social response to the disabled person that 'disables' as much, if not more so than, the impairment itself. (Thompson, 2011: 114)

It is significant that people with disabilities are more likely than others to experience social disadvantage, low socioeconomic status and inadequate social support which are also major risk factors for mental illness (Jenkins and Rigg, 2004).

Traditional attitudes towards people with a disability have tended to medicalise the disability. If disability is seen as damage to the body, it then requires diagnosis and treatment which places problems within the individual whilst ignoring the wider social dimension of discrimination. Efforts go into trying to make disabled people more comfortable and able to cope with their impairment, both physically and emotionally, rather than into ensuring that the social and physical barriers are removed and people's attitudes are challenged. In describing the efforts that health or education professionals go to minimise or eliminate the impairment, Middleton (1996: 37) writes:

> All these efforts to make a child normal by stimulating brain waves, hanging them upside down, pushing, pulling, cajoling, mean that the child receives the very clear message that there is something about them that nobody likes. Chances are that

they will learn to not like it either. Since it is likely to be something about which, realistically they can do little or nothing about, this over-emphasis is likely only to create a sense of failure or even self-hate.

Attitudes towards disability can be demeaning, reinforcing negative images and perceptions and assuming that disabled young people are helpless and dependent rather than people with rights and strengths. Wilson (2003) suggests that one of the major causes of emotional distress for disabled people is not their physical impairment but the effect that it has on their relationships and their ability to manage their environment. A disabled child's experience is often characterised by a mismatch between their actual needs and their needs as perceived by their carers. This gap can lead either to over-care which places unnecessary restrictions on their freedom or to under-care, perhaps to the point of neglect (Wilson, 2003: 114).

These attitudes and beliefs about disability single disabled children out as a group deserving of our compassion and pity and unfortunately contempt. Disability acts as a social division, cutting young people off from the mainstream and causing them to feel isolated and oppressed and therefore particularly vulnerable to low self-esteem, a distorted sense of self and to mental illness.

Practitioners working with disabled children and young people who have mental health problems need to be aware of these negative attitudes and rather than focusing on compassion, focus on ways of empowering children and young people with disabilities to feel positive about themselves as individuals and have a strong sense of identity. It is also essential to consider the other barriers to accessing services such as physical access and a lack of understanding of mental health workers about disability issues. It is therefore important for mental health services to be 'disability friendly'. Furthermore, disability workers and others coming into contact with young people with disabilities should be proactive in liaising with and referring people with disabilities to mental health services rather than assuming that problems with adjustment to disability are inevitable or will improve with time (Honey et al., 2013).

CURRENT ANTI-DISCRIMINATORY LEGISLATION

So far this chapter has explored the meaning and impact of values, attitudes, beliefs and inequalities on children, young people and their families. It has reflected on ways that individuals can challenge their own values and beliefs to gain greater awareness of how they impact on children and young people. As Thompson's PCS analysis suggests, challenging discrimination at an individual level is difficult to do if it is not linked to practice at both a cultural and structural level. Legislation at an international, national and local level needs to underpin all anti-discriminatory practice and guide organisations and practitioners in their approach to working with all children, adolescents and families.

The United Nations Convention on the Rights of the Child (1989)

It is difficult to write about issues around equality and inequality in relation to children and young people without acknowledging that children themselves, regardless of race, religion, disability, gender or culture, are often discriminated against and their rights disregarded by adults who believe they know what is best. Children's rights were touched upon in Chapter 3 with some case studies, and it is relevant to mention children's rights again here in relation to values. The United Nations Convention on the Rights of the Child (UNCRC, 1989) is an international human rights treaty that grants all children and young people (aged 17 and under) a comprehensive set of rights. The UK signed the Convention on 19 April 1990, ratified it on 16 December 1991 and it came into force on 15 January 1992. It is interesting to note, however, that the UK exercised a reservation on Article 22 until 2008. Article 22 relates to children having the right to special protection and help if they are refugees (if they have been forced to leave their home and live in another country) as well as all the other rights in the Convention. Immigration and nationality matters took precedence over the interests of children, effectively leading to a disregard for Articles 2 (non-discrimination of children), 3 (best interest) and 12 (respect for the child's views) (Ayotte and Williamson, 2001). Once the reservation was finally withdrawn asylum seeking and trafficked children were afforded the same rights as other children in Britain to health, education and other support services (UNICEF, 2008).

The UNCRC is presently the most widely ratified international human rights treaty. It is the only international human rights treaty to include civil, political, economic, social and cultural rights. It sets out in detail what every child needs to have a safe, happy and fulfilled childhood regardless of their sex, religion, social origin and where and to whom they were born. The Convention gives children and young people over 40 rights, including the right to:

- Special protection measures and assistance.
- Access to services such as education and health care.
- Develop their personalities, abilities and talents to the fullest potential.
- Grow up in an environment of happiness, love and understanding.
- Be informed about and participate in achieving their rights in an accessible and active manner.

The UNCRC gives all organisations a framework within which to ensure that all children are heard. On a national level, legislation is needed to ensure that this happens and that particular groups of people are not marginalised or discriminated against.

The Equality Act 2010

The Equality Act 2010 provides a single legal framework with clear, streamlined law to more effectively tackle disadvantage and discrimination. It brings together over

116 separate pieces of legislation into one single Act. Combined, they make up a new Act that provides a legal framework to protect the rights of individuals and advance equality of opportunity for all.

It also makes the law stronger in some areas. It has created a Single Public Sector Equality Duty which covers eight protected characteristics:

- Age
- Disability
- Gender reassignment
- Pregnancy and maternity
- Race
- Religion and belief
- Sex
- Sexual orientation.

Not only do public and private bodies have a duty to protect the rights of people with protected characteristics and ensure that they are not discriminated against but they have to be more proactive and to go beyond non-discrimination by advancing equality. Under the general duty, in Section 149 of the Equality Act, all public bodies need to have due regard to:

(a) Eliminate discrimination, harassment, victimisation and any other conduct prohibited by the Act;
(b) Advance equality of opportunity between people who share a relevant protected characteristic and people who do not share it;
(c) Foster good relations between people who share a relevant protected characteristic and people who do not share it.

This is particularly important in schools and services for children and young people who are starting out in life and establishing their individuality and identity. It supports every child's right to grow up free of discrimination and improves each child's access to the five outcomes of *Every Child Matters* (Department for Education and Skills, 2003).

STRATEGIES TO COMBAT AND PROMOTE ANTI-DISCRIMINATORY PRACTICE

Brinley Harper and Dwivedi (2004) suggest that culturally competent services for children and young people should be embedded in meaningful, appropriate policy frameworks. Legislation such as the Equality Act provides a framework so that services and organisations can plan, develop and deliver policies and services that promote equality and are culturally sensitive. They suggest that there should be active community involvement at both an individual and organisational level. Staff should be well educated in issues around cultural sensitivity and diversity and should receive regular and up to date training. There should also be a focus on supportive and sensitive administrative and clinical practices which take account of cultural identity. Dwivedi (1996, cited in Brinley Harper and Dwivedi, 2004) gives further guidance on how to ensure that services engage in anti-discriminatory practice. He writes about the importance of setting up community outreach work and interpreter and translation services which ensure that 'subjugated narratives' are heard. In relation to professional development he states that it:

> ... needs to incorporate the perspective of difference and diversity aiming not only to raise cultural awareness by gaining knowledge but also cultural sensitivity through experiences that challenge one's respective cultural identities and their influence on understanding and acceptance of others. (p. 6)

As a starting point for any child or young person who we meet in a professional capacity we need to ensure that we have considered their wider context and the meanings that they have made of their experiences. It is only when we have considered multiple perspectives that we can see whether our perspective makes any sense to them. Dogra (2004: 241) suggests the following key areas that the practitioner needs to know about the child and their family:

- Who is the child and what constitutes their life? What are their interests, important relationships and main concerns?
- What does the child expect from the practitioner? What are the child's values and fears? What does the child hope to accomplish in the visit or over the longer term?
- How does the child experience their problems?
- What are the child's ideas about the problem?
- What are the child's main feelings about the problem?

Child-centred questioning focuses on the sense that they make of the issues to ensure that the approach is culturally appropriate and to take into account their context and individual perspective. It is important to explore the child and their family's own meanings of mental health and to avoid making assumptions or trying to explain things in a way that fits with your own values and beliefs.

HOW ANTI-DISCRIMINATORY LEGISLATION AND PRACTICE CAN MAKE A DIFFERENCE

Promoting the equality of lesbian, gay, bisexual and transgender (LGBT) young people

One of the most significant implications of the Equality Act 2010 is that it highlights the importance of ensuring equality for people based on their sexual orientation or gender identity. LGBT young people are more at risk of developing mental health problems than their heterosexual peers; 23% of lesbian, gay and bisexual young people have tried to kill themselves and 56% have self-harmed (Guasp, 2012). Figures from Stonewall show that in the past year 3% of gay and bisexual men have attempted suicide (Guasp, 2012). These figures show how essential it is that schools, health and youth services promote equality for young LGBT people. *No Health Without Mental Health* (Department of Health, 2011) states that 'People who are lesbian, gay and bisexual all have a higher risk of mental health problems and of self-harm. They also suffer more attacks and violence. Experiences of mental health services are reportedly poor, and monitoring of sexual orientation is patchy, making it less easy to develop tailored service responses.' Discrimination of LGBT young people is particularly disproportionate because it is so prevalent in our society and frequently occurs within families where parents reject their child because of their sexual orientation. The emotional impact of this on the child is huge.

The Equality Act 2010 requires that public services actively promote equality and this has a potentially huge impact on children, young people and families who are LGBT. Section 28 of the Local Government Act 1988 stated that a local authority:

> ... shall not intentionally promote homosexuality or publish material with the inten- tion of promoting homosexuality ... [or] promote the teaching in any maintained school of the acceptability of homosexuality as a pretended family relationship.

This was repealed in 2000 in Scotland and in 2003 in the rest of Great Britain by Section 122 of the Local Government Act 2003. This prejudice and discrimi- nation supported homophobia and homophobic bullying at a national level and made it almost impossible for schools and public services to challenge discrim- ination on the grounds of sexuality and gender identity. *The School Report* (Guasp, 2012), produced by the national campaign group Stonewall in conjunc- tion with Cambridge University, reveals the extent of homophobic bullying in schools. The report shows how the work done to challenge homophobic atti- tudes has improved the lives of LGBT young people since the repeal of Section 28. It is encouraging to see that levels of homophobic bullying have fallen by 10% since 2007 and the number of schools saying that homophobic bullying is wrong has more than doubled, to 50%. However, prejudice and homophobic bullying are still far too prevalent in schools in the UK and *The School Report* states that:

> More than half of lesbian, gay and bisexual young people still report experiencing homophobic bullying and its damaging impact is just as pronounced. Over two in five gay pupils who experience homophobic bullying attempt or think about taking their own life as a direct consequence. Three in five young people say that bully- ing has a direct impact on their school work and straight-A students have told us it makes them want to leave education entirely. As policymakers look for ways to boost attainment and raise aspiration it's clear that tackling homophobic bullying should be close to the top of their agenda. (Guasp, 2012: 3)

Schools need to take active steps to prevent and respond to homophobic bullying and discrimination. It is notable that only half of lesbian, gay and bisexual pupils report that their schools say homophobic bullying is wrong. In comparison, 95% of schools say bullying because of ethnicity is wrong and 90% say bullying because of disability is wrong. Schools that positively address and teach about gay people and issues are far more likely to reduce homophobic bullying and create a positive learning environment for lesbian, gay and bisexual pupils.

A positive learning environment and anti-homophobic message can be created in schools in some of the following ways:

- Whole school training.
- Changing and publicising policy and raising awareness through posters and clear communication to pupils, staff and parents.
- Letting pupils know that if they experience homophobic bullying, they will be supported and incidents will be taken seriously.
- Celebrating LGBT History Month.
- Delivering lessons with an LGBT theme.
- Stocking a range of books with LGBT themes.
- Role model visits.

Mental health services too need to address the particular needs of LGBT young people, who are often reluctant to access services because of the stigma of mental illness, being gay or both. Accessibility, flexibility and client-centred services are more likely to address the needs of young people who have already experienced high levels of discrimination and prejudice.

CONCLUSION

This short chapter has attempted to introduce those working with children, young people and their families to the complexities of working ethically and in a culturally competent way. It has emphasised the importance of practitioners having a clear awareness of their own world views and the ability to take into account the world view of their clients. It also points out that we must consider the systematic oppression that certain groups that have lived with whilst other groups have benefitted from the inherent privileges of their ethnicity, gender and class.

REFERENCES

Adiche, C. (2009) *The Dangers of the Single Story*. Available from: www.ted.com/talks/chimamanda_adichie_the_danger_of_a_single_story.html?source=email#.UZJiQxnd-6J.gmail. (accessed 21 May 2013).

Allport, G. (1954) *The Nature of Prejudice*. Boston, MA: Beacon Press.

Association of American Medical Colleges (1999) *Report III: Contemporary Issues in Medicine*. Washington, DC: Communication in Medicine.

Ayotte, W. and Williamson, L. (2001) *Separated Children in the UK: An Overview of the Current Situation*. Available from: www.refugeecouncil.org.uk/latest/news/1102_refugee_children_arriving_alone_are_being_left_unsupported_and_unprotected_reveals_uk_repor (accessed September 2013).

Banhatti, R. and Bhate, S. (2002) Mental Health Needs of Ethnic Minority Children. In Dwivedi, K.N. (ed.) *Meeting the Needs of Ethnic Minority Children*, 2nd edn. London: Jessica Kingsley, pp. 66–90.

Beauchamp, T. and Childress, J. (2001) *Principles of Biomedical Ethics*, 5th edn. New York: Oxford University Press.

Brinley Harper, P. and Dwivedi, R. (2004) Developing Culturally Sensitive Services to Meet the Mental Health Needs of Ethnic Minority Children. In Dwivedi, K.N. and Brinley Harper, P. (eds) *Promoting the Emotional Well-being of Children and Adolescents and Preventing Their Mental Ill Health: A Handbook*. London: Jessica Kingsley, pp. 234–55.

Burnham, J., Palma, D. and Whitehouse, L. (2008) Learning as a Context for Differences and Differences as a Context for Learning. *Journal of Family Therapy*, 30(4): 529–42.

Cecchin, G. (1987) Hypothesising, Circularity and Neutrality Revisited: An Invitation to Curiosity. *Family Process*, 26 (4): 405–13.

Coleman, J. (2011) *The Nature of Adolescence*. Hove: Routledge.

Cuthbert, S. and Quallington, J. (2008) *Values for Care Practice*. Exeter: Reflect Press.

Davies, S. (2013) Calls for Changes after Worcester Path Branded 'Unusable' for Wheelchair Users. *Worcester News*, 21 August. Available from: www.worcesternews.co.uk/news/10625057. Worcester_path_branded__unusable__for_wheelchairs/ (accessed September 2013).

Department for Education and Skills (2003) *Every Child Matters*. Available from: webarchive. nationalarchives.gov.uk/20130401151715/https://www.education.gov.uk/publications/eOrderingDownload/ECM-Summary.pdf (accessed September 2013).

Department of Health (2011) *No Health Without Mental Health*. Available from: www. dh.gov.uk/en/Publicationsandstatistics/Publications/PublicationsPolicyAndGuidance/DH_123766 (accessed October 2012).

Dogra, N. (2004) Child Psychiatry Selection. *Child and Adolescent Mental Health*, 9 (1): 40–41.

Dogra, N. (2007) Cultural Diversity in Working with Vulnerable Children. In Vostanis, P. (ed.) *Mental Health Interventions and Services for Vulnerable Children and Young People*. London: Jessica Kingsley, pp. 235–45.

Dwivedi, K.N. and Brinley Harper, P. (eds) (2004) *Promoting the Emotional Well-being of Children and Adolescents and Preventing Their Mental Ill Health: A Handbook*. London: Jessica Kingsley.

Equality Act (2010) London: TSO/Equality & Human Rights Commission. Available from: www.equalityhumanrights.com/legal-and-policy/equality-act/ (accessed September 2013).

Guasp, A. (2012) *The School Report: The Experiences of Gay Young People in Britain's Schools in 2012*. University of Cambridge and Stonewall. Available from: www.stonewall. org.uk/atschool (accessed September 2013).

Halson, A. (2005) White – British or Not. *Context*, 80: 35–6.

Hills, J., Brewer, M., Jenkins, S., Lister, R., Lupron, R., Machin, S., Mills, C., Modood, T., Rees, T. and Riddell, S. (2010) *An Anatomy of Economic Inequality in the UK: Report of the National Equality Panel*. London: Government Equalities Office.

Honey, A., Emerson, E., Llewellyn, G. and Kariuki, M. (2013) Mental Health and Disability. In Stone, J.H. and Blouin, M. (eds) *International Encyclopedia of Rehabilitation*. Available from: cirrie.buffalo.edu/encyclopedia/en/article/305/ (accessed September 2013).

Jasper, M. (2003) *Beginning Reflective Practice*. Cheltenham: Nelson Thornes.

Jenkins, S. and Rigg, J. (2004). Disability and Disadvantage: Selection, Onset and Duration Effects. *Journal of Social Policy*, 33 (3): 479–501.

Lau, A. (1994) Gender, Culture and Family Life. *Context*, 20: 7–10.

Local Government Act (1988) Available from: www.legislation.gov.uk/ukpga/1988/9/contents (accessed March 2013).

Local Government Act (2003) Available from: www.legislation.gov.uk/ukpga/2003/26/pdfs/ ukpga_20030026_en.pdf (accessed on 4 March 2013).

Mental Health Foundation (2013) *Black and Ethnic Minority Communities*. Available from: www.mentalhealth.org.uk/help-information/mental-health-a-z/B/BME-communities/ (accessed on 15 July 2013).

Middleton, L. (1996) *Making a Difference: Social Work with Disabled Children*. New York: Venture Press.

Phibbs, H. (2009) It is Not Racist to State that Gypsy Camps Frequently Cause an Increase in Crime and Mess – It is a Statement of Fact. *The Daily Mail Online*, 5 January. Available from: www.dailymail.co.uk/debate/article-1105510/It-racist-state-gypsy-camps-frequently-cause-increase-crime-mess--statement-fact.html (accessed September 2013).

Salway, S., Turner, D., Ghazala, M., Carter, L., Skinner, J., Bostan, B., Gerrish, K. and Ellison, G. (2013) *High Quality Health Care Commissioning: Why Race Equality Must be at its Heart*. Race Equality Foundation. Available from: www.better-health.org.uk/sites/default/files/ briefings/downloads/High%20quality%20healthcare%20commissioning-%20format2.pdf (accessed 4 September 2013).

Savill, R. (2002) Bristol: 'These Kids Will Nick Anything for Drugs'. *The Daily Telegraph*, 2 November. Available from: www.telegraph.co.uk/news/uknews/1411948/Bristol-These-kids-will-nick-anything-for-drugs.html (accessed September 2013).

Smith, H.C. (2008) Bridging the Gap: Therapy through Interpreters. *Therapy Today*, 19 (6): 21–3.

Thompson, N. (2006) *Anti-discriminatory Practice*, 4th edn. Basingstoke: Palgrave Macmillan.

Thompson, N. (2011) *Promoting Equality*. Basingstoke: Palgrave Macmillan.

UNICEF, (2008) *A Summary of the UN Convention on the Rights of the Child*. Available at: www.unicef.org.uk/Documents/Publication-pdfs/betterlifeleaflet2012_press.pdf (accessed on 7 November 2013).

UNCRC (1989) United Nations Convention on the Rights of the Child. Available from: www.education.gov.uk/childrenandyoungpeople/healthandwellbeing/b0074766/uncrc. (accessed on 4.3.2013).

Walker, B.A. (1994) Valuing Differences: The Concept and a Model. In Mabey, C. and Iles, P. (eds) *Managing Learning*. London: Routledge, pp. 211–23.

Webb, R. and Tossell, D. (1999) *Social Issues for Carers*. London: Arnold.

Wilkinson, R. and Pickett, K. (2009) *The Spirit Level: Why More Equal Societies Almost Always Do Better*. London: Allen Lane.

Wilson, A. (2003) 'Real Jobs', 'Learning Difficulties' and 'Supported Employment'. *Disability and Society*, 18 (2): 99–115.

INDEX

Lightning Source UK Ltd.
Milton Keynes UK
UKOW07f2301220915

259091UK00004B/209/P

9 781446 249451